CARING FOR THE
DYING

Contemporary Issues

Series Editors: Robert M. Baird
Stuart E. Rosenbaum

Volumes edited by Robert M. Baird and Stuart E. Rosenbaum
unless otherwise noted.

CARING FOR THE
DYING

critical issues
at the edge of life

edited by

ROBERT M. BAIRD
& STUART E. ROSENBAUM

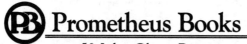 **Prometheus Books**

59 John Glenn Drive
Amherst, New York 14228-2197

Published 2003 by Prometheus Books

Inquiries should be addressed to
Prometheus Books
59 John Glenn Drive
Amherst, New York 14228–2197

716–691–0133 (x207). FAX: 716–564–2711.
WWW.PROMETHEUSBOOKS.COM

07 06 05 04 03   5 4 3 2 1

Library of Congress Cataloging-in-Publication Data

Caring for the dying : critical issues at the edge of life / edited by Robert M.
    Baird and Stuart E. Rosenbaum.
        p.   cm. — (Contemporary Issues series)
    Includes bibliographical references.
    ISBN 1-57392-969-7 (alk. paper)
    1. Terminal care. 2. Palliative treatment. 3. Death—Psychological
aspects. I. Baird, Robert M., 1937– II. Rosenbaum, Stuart E.
III. Contemporary Issues (Amherst, N.Y.)

R726.8 .C385 2002
362.1'75—dc21   2002068058

Printed in the United States of America on acid-free paper

CONTENTS

PART THREE: SPIRITUAL CARING FOR THE DYING

PART FOUR: LEGAL ISSUES AT THE END OF LIFE

INTRODUCTION

Robert M. Baird and
Stuart E. Rosenbaum

A hospital chaplain was mentoring a young minister. A few weeks into the minister's training, a woman, quite agitated, came to the chaplain's office. She reported to the two of them that her husband had just been told that he was terminally ill. This was especially disturbing to her, she said, because her husband was "not a Christian." She wanted a minister to go to his hospital room and "convert him." "Nothing else matters," she said. "That's really the only need he has now—the need to become a Christian." Having received assurance that a minister would visit her husband, she departed. The chaplain asked the minister-in-training if he would be willing to see the patient. When the young minister agreed, the chaplain inquired, "What do you think you can do for that man? What role can you play in his life? What do you think his needs *really* are?" The chaplain used this and other experiences to help the young minister understand that regardless of what anybody else says a person has need of, only the person himself or herself is truly in a position to reveal those needs. A cardinal principle of caring is that one should avoid entering relationships with others with rigid presuppositions about their needs. The first responsibility in any caring relationship is to be open to others in a way that encourages others to reveal freely what their needs genuinely are. Only then can an appropriate and responsible response be made.

People face death and dying differently; consequently, end-of-life needs vary. Awareness of this is crucial for both the dying and for those caring for the dying. This is an underlying theme of the essays in this volume. The purpose of this introduction is to reinforce this crucial principle of effective caring by briefly examining several philosophical reflections on the variety of ways individuals confront death and dying. This will serve as a helpful framework for reading and reflecting on these essays.

The philosopher Martin Heidegger in his work *Being and Time* distinguishes two prominent responses to death and dying. The tendency of many is to deny the personal reality of death altogether. Of course, in one sense, notes Heidegger, death cannot be denied; it is a reality constantly surrounding us. People are dying all the time. But the human capacity for self-deception is enormous, particularly with regard to death and dying. People can be heard to say, "One of these days one will die too; but right now it has nothing to do with [me]."[1] According to Heidegger, the reality of death is often denied by allocating it to the indefinite future of the indefinite "one."

Leo Tolstoy in *The Death of Ivan Ilych* captures this attitude. The death of Ivan "aroused, as usual, in all who heard of it the complacent feeling that, 'it is he who is dead and not I.' Each one thought or felt, 'Well, he's dead but I'm alive.' "[2] Upon viewing Ivan's body, Peter Ivanovich, a friend of Ivan's, thought that Ivan's dead face expressed a warning, but Peter was convinced that the warning was "at least not applicable to him."[3] Momentarily terrified at the thought that what happened to Ivan might also happen to him, Peter consoled himself with "the customary reflection . . . that this had happened to Ivan Ilych and not to him, and that it should not and could not happen to him, and that to think that it could would be yielding to depression which he ought not to do."[4] At the service Peter "did not look once at the dead man, did not yield to any depressing influence, and was one of the first to leave the room."[5] Of course, Peter and the others were only going through the same form of self-deception that Ivan himself had earlier attempted. The syllogism Ivan had learned: " 'Caius is a man, men are mortal, therefore Caius is mortal,' had always seemed to him correct as applied to Caius, but certainly not as applied to himself. That Caius—man in the abstract—was mortal, was perfectly correct, but he was not Caius, not an abstract man, but a creature quite, quite separate from the others. . . .' Caius really was mortal, and it was right for him to die; but for me, little Vanya, Ivan Ilych, with all my thoughts and emotions, it's altogether a different matter. It cannot be that I ought to die.' "[6]

On the other hand, says Heidegger, some individuals look death in the face, taking it for what it is, a boundary beyond which one cannot go. Moreover, this intense awareness that life is limited gives rise to a creative use of the time remaining. Heidegger so admires this reaction that he encourages individuals to live, thoroughly conscious of one's own impending death, of one's own inevitable confrontation with nothingness. For such an awareness or consciousness can give rise to a life that refuses to "while away" time with trivia, in a life that creatively "gets on" with crucial matters.

Still another way of confronting death is suggested by Jean-Paul Sartre in his short story "The Wall." Pablo Ibbieta, a political prisoner, is sentenced to die. "I'd never thought about death," he reflects, "because I never had any reason to, but now the reason was here and there was nothing to do but think about it."[7] Pablo discovers death to be a wall beyond which one cannot go, a wall beyond which Pablo cannot even mentally project himself. Repeatedly the point is made that one who knows he is going to die is different from one who is not confronted with imminent death, and the fundamental difference is that the living can "think about tomorrow."[8] For the dying, "as soon as I tried to think of anything else I saw rifle barrels pointing at me."[9]

The significance of this difference between the living and the imminently dying is the breakdown in communication between the two. Thinking about his girl Concha, Pablo says: "I had no more desire to see her, I had nothing more to say to her. . . . If she looked at me now, the look would stay in her eyes, it wouldn't reach me. I was alone."[10] The dying person is often alone, for frequently he cannot communicate with the living. A fundamental characteristic of the living is to project into the not-yet, to live mentally in the future. But this is precisely what the dying man, affirms Sartre in "The Wall," cannot do. He is confined to the now, the present moment, hemmed in by the barrier of death. The living and the imminently dying, therefore, live in different worlds. For the living, eyes are focused on the future. For the dying, anticipation of death has eliminated the future. Communication between the two may become virtually impossible.

Tolstoy in *The Death of Ivan Ilych* also captures this difficulty in communication. When Ivan received the disturbing news from his doctor, he went home and "began to tell his wife about it. She listened, but in the middle of his account his daughter came in with her hat on, ready to go out with her mother. She sat down reluctantly to listen to this tedious story, but could not stand it long, and her mother too did not hear him to the end."[11] Ivan could no longer deceive himself: "something terrible, new, and more important than anything before in his life, was taking place within him of which he alone was aware. Those about him did not understand or would not understand it, but thought everything in the world was going on as usual. That tormented Ivan Ilych more than anything."[12] Ivan "had to live thus on the brink of an abyss, with no one who understood."[13] And so of his dying Ivan concluded: "Why speak of it? She won't understand."[14]

Paul Tillich, in *The Courage to Be*, also describes individuals' differing experiences with death. For many, the confrontation with death is the encounter with nonbeing. The confrontation involved is not simply an abstract or intellectual acknowledgment of death, but rather an existential awareness at the feeling level that "nonbeing is a part of one's own being."[15] Death is not a reality laying plans for an ambush somewhere out in the future; it is a constant companion. From the moment of birth, one is in the process of dying. Nothingness, nonbeing, death is an ever-stalking threat waiting for that decisive point in time when it brutally hurls the living soul "out of existence."[16] This awareness that one must die is, for Tillich, the root of all anxiety. Anxiety is defined as "the state in which a being is aware of its possible nonbeing."[17] Anxiety is the "gut" recognition that in the last analysis one is going to die and there is nothing to be done about it. How can one defend oneself against this nothingness? The magnitude of the anxiety produced by the awareness that one is finally helpless "to preserve one's own being . . ."[18] is beyond parallel. Such anxiety can never be eliminated; it is a part of the structure of human existence.

Tolstoy's Ivan experiences this anxiety. At the moment when the meaning of death broke through to Ivan, his "heart sank and he felt dazed. 'My God! My God!' he muttered. . . . It's not a question of appendix or kidney, but of life and . . . death. . . . I'm dying. . . . There was light and now there is darkness. I was here and now I am going there! Where? . . . When I am not, what will there be? There will be nothing. Then where shall I be when I am no more?"[19] Eventually when the finality of it took hold of him, Ivan began a screaming "that continued for three days, and was so terrible that one could not hear it through two closed doors without horror."[20]

The question for Tillich becomes: Is there the possibility of affirming oneself in the face of the threat of nonbeing? Is there the possibility for the courage to be? His answer is yes. At this point his religious commitment comes in to play, as it does for many individuals confronting death. Courage is defined by Tillich as "the self-affirmation of being in spite of nonbeing."[21] For Tillich, this courage to be or this self-affirmation is expressed in three interrelated ways. First, instead of being overcome by despair in the face of death, those who have the courage to be affirm themselves as incomparably valuable and unique individuals, free to have a determinative influence in spite of the impending death. Second, instead of being overwhelmed by anxiety in the encounter with death, those who have the courage to be affirm themselves as meaningful participants in the various communities of which they are a part. Finally, and most important, instead of yielding to the horror of the threatened nothingness, those who have the courage to be affirm by faith (which always involves a daring risk) the power of God. Entailed by this is nothing less than the faith affirmation that "the ground of everything that is . . . is living creativity . . . [which is] eternally conquering its own nonbeing."[22] All of which is to say that God or being-itself is also faced with nonbeing, but in its power is continually overcoming the threat. The person of faith participates in this overcoming. Indeed, Tillich argues that every instance of finite courage to be (whether recognized by the individual or not) has its source in the power of being-itself to overcome its nemesis, nonbeing. By affirming our being we participate in the self-affirmation of being-itself. There are no valid arguments for the "existence" of God, but there are acts of courage in which we affirm the power of being, whether we know it or not.

Ivan Ilych "caught sight of the light. . . . And suddenly . . . what had been oppressing him and would not leave him was all dropping away at once from two sides, from ten sides, from all sides. . . . There was no fear because there was no death. In place of death was light. 'So that's what it is!' he suddenly exclaimed aloud. 'What joy!' To him all this happened in a single instant. . . . For those present his agony continued for another two hours. . . . Something rattled in his throat, his emaciated body twitched. . . . 'It is finished!' said someone near him. . . . 'Death is finished,' he said to himself. 'It is no more!' He drew in a breath, stopped in the midst of a sigh, stretched out, and died."[23]

These existential analyses of confrontation with death are

provocative. For present purposes, the point to be emphasized is that all of these descriptions are valuable as portraits of different ways people encounter death. There are those who refuse to face death by disguising its reality; those who acknowledge death's reality in a way that frees or liberates them to deal creatively with the life remaining; those who confront death as a Sartrean "encounter with a wall," experiencing an inability to communicate with those around them who are continuing to project into the future; those whose dying generates hopeless anxiety; and those who overcome death by the courage to be, that is, by faith they affirm and thereby participate in what Tillich calls the power of being-itself (God) to overcome nonbeing (death).

The overwhelmingly important conclusion to be derived is this: in any caring relationship with one who is dying, the first responsibility is to be open to individuals in order that they may be permitted the luxury of revealing where they are in terms of their present attitude toward death. As indicated, this serves as an unstated theme of most of the essays comprising this collection.

PART ONE: THE HOSPICE MOVEMENT

The first section of this book focuses on the hospice movement. One consequence of the ongoing controversy over euthanasia[24] and the legalization of physician-assisted suicide in Oregon has been renewed concern for more adequate end-of-life care. Since hospice is that institution solely devoted to such care, increasing interest in hospice is emerging nationally. It is as if the specter of euthanasia and physician-assisted suicide have encouraged deeper reflection on end-of-life issues and on the possibilities of providing the kind of comfort and support to those who are dying that would render moot the question of suicide. The initial essay in this section is by Naomi Naierman, president and CEO of the American Hospice Foundation. Motivated by the unfortunate fact that hospice is still a mystery to many people, she makes clear the nature of hospice and debunks ten common hospice myths. The second selection provides both a brief history of the hospice movement and a comparison of hospice activities in England, where the modern hospice movement began, and the United States. The authors of the second selection also discuss the funding of hospice care by Medicare.

When decisions are made in the intensive care unit to withdraw treatment as a means of allowing the patient to die, hospice principles are relevant. The difficulty is that hospice guidelines were developed primarily for care of those dying at home. Implementing the "hospice game of terminal care" in a different setting is, according to Helen Chapple, comparable to playing baseball on a football field. She divides the process in the intensive care unit into two segments: the period between deciding to withdraw treatment and the actual withdrawal, and the period between withdrawal and death. Caring guidelines are suggested for each period. Her remarks are addressed to nurses, but are useful for any caring companion.

"Beyond 'Death with Dignity': A Hospice Vignette," written by a hospice social worker with fifteen years experience, is brief, disturbing in some of its details, and emphatic about the importance of timely hospice intervention. The concluding selection by Bruce Chamberlain addresses the problem that the word *hospice* connotes to many people: "giving up, failure, and imminent death." Some who are concerned about this image have even suggested that the term *hospice* should be replaced by "end-of-life care" or "palliative care," but Chamberlain rejects this suggestion because he sees the problem as systemic. The image problem would, therefore, carry over to whatever name was used if the problems in the system are not rectified. He is specifically concerned that too many hospice programs do not provide the array of services that the Medicare Hospice Benefit program makes available, and in failing to do so have failed to communicate to the public a positive image of hospice.

PART TWO: PALLIATIVE CARE AT THE END OF LIFE

A major concern for individuals confronting dying is pain. The essays in this section focus on palliative care, the holistic care of patients whose life expectancy is limited. The aim of such comprehensive care is to enhance the quality of life at the end of life by alleviating physical pain and emotional distress. The initial selection by Clyde Nabe is a detailed analysis of human suffering. Precisely when and to what extent suffering should be alleviated depends on the value or disvalue associated with such suffering, normally as determined by the one who is suffering. Nabe argues that suffering in and of itself is evil, but acknowledges that suffering can, under some circumstances, be a means to a desirable end. The burden of proof, however, always rests with the one who maintains that suffering is worthwhile. Again, being clear about this matter is crucial both for the one who is suffering and for the caregiver.

The essay by Quill, Lee, and Nunn focuses on the challenging issues for palliative care in the case of terminally ill patients who are "ready to die." Five modes of palliative intervention are described "in order of increasing legal and ethical uncertainty." This account is followed by an analysis of five clinical cases illustrating when each of the five intervention modes might be justified.

One of the keys, of course, to effective palliative care is the use of drugs to control pain. Both because they are legitimately used to terminate life under certain circumstances[25] and because they can incidentally cause death, the use of drugs in pain control has recently become a controversial political issue. The focus of this controversy is the Pain Relief Promotion Act of 1999. Passed in the U.S. House of Representatives, it is now being considered by the Senate. Many see the act as ultimately aimed at reversing the Oregon decision to permit physician-assisted suicide. Many who oppose physician-assisted suicide, however, are concerned that the effect of the bill will be to limit the aggressive treatment of pain by physicians and hospice personnel. This controversy is the subject of the next three essays in this section. The editorial by Marcia Angell from the *New England Journal of Medicine* provides a good introduction to this controversy and also expresses a political position with regard to legislation pending in Congress. This piece is followed by two essays taken from congressional testimony on the Pain Relief Promotion Act of 1999.

The two concluding essays in this section focus on palliative sedation, the act of keeping a patient in a sedated or unconscious state as a way of managing pain that cannot otherwise be controlled. In the first of these pieces, Paul Rousseau advances a definition of palliative sedation, discusses its use for both physical and existential suffering, and focuses on the latter by providing guidelines for the use of palliative sedation in cases of existential suffering. Clay Jackson's brief essay is a positive response to Rousseau, commending Rousseau for use of the phrase "palliative sedation" rather than the frequently used "terminal sedation." The latter is ambiguous and fails to make clear that the purpose of such sedation is the relief of suffering, not the termination of life.

PART THREE: SPIRITUAL CARING FOR THE DYING

The intent of the articles in this section is captured by the opening paragraph of the lead essay by Myles Sheehan: "What does it mean to attend to the spiritual needs of patients as they face serious illness? And what, if any, impact does a person's spirituality have on choices at the end of life? Does the openness of caregivers to a patent's spiritual experience affect their interaction with patients? Could explicit attention to spirituality help doctors and patients be frank about the goals of treatment and a person's choices about therapy?" Sheehan proceeds to define spirituality and to advance reasons why physicians, in particular, should be concerned with spirituality.

In "Spiritual Care at the End of Life," Tad Dunne provides an inclusive understanding of the spiritual that would be relevant for patients who are religious in the traditional sense and to those who are not. He focuses on the spiritual as one's concern with ultimate meaning. Influenced by Bernard Lonergan's analysis of faith, hope, and love and providing his own interpretation of these spiritual categories, Dunne makes specific suggestions for caregivers as they provide spiritual care at the end of life.

The essay by Redding, "Control Theory in Dying: What Do We Know?" explicitly emphasizes the point made in the beginning of this introduction. "The only person who can inform us, on an existential level, of what is needed at the end of life is the individual who is dying." For many patients, she notes, the matter of control in the dying process is crucial to giving meaning to the event.

We often speak of a "good" death. In fact, the word *euthanasia* is derived from the Greek *eu thanatos* meaning "good death." But what are the components of such a death? The article "In Search of a Good Death: Observations of Patients, Families, and Providers" reports on a study designed to answer this question. Participants in the study included physicians, nurses, chaplains, social workers, hospice volunteers, patients, and families of patients. Six components of a good death emerged in the study, each of which is discussed in the essay.

The concluding essay is quite narrow in focus: withholding nutrition and hydration from a terminal Jewish patient. It illustrates clearly the importance of taking into account the religious traditions of individuals in the care of the dying.

PART FOUR: LEGAL ISSUES AT THE END OF LIFE: ADVANCE DIRECTIVES

Ann Alpert and Bernard Lo introduce scenarios based on actual cases as a way of introducing the difficulties that can arise between a patient's family serving as proxy for the patient and the physician, particularly when the medical situation of the patient takes an unexpected turn. Practical suggestions are made for attempting to negotiate these conflicts. The legal issues involved in these situations can create considerable anxiety for the attending physician. Marshall Kapp's essay, "Anxieties as a Legal Impediment to the Doctor-Proxy Relationship," addresses this issue and proposes strategies for addressing some of the problems that arise. Sensitivity to these issues is important for physician, patient, and proxy.

In advanced directives, such as the durable power of attorney, legal rights are granted to proxies and a contract is created. Joseph Fins maintains that complementing the contractual relationship that is established with a covenant view of the patient-proxy relationship can often enhance the quality of advance-care planning. While not every patient has the opportunity to be represented by a proxy with whom a covenantal relationship is possible, when it is possible, argues Fins, wise decisions in complex medical circumstances become more likely.

The concluding article by Norman Cantor is a review of the present state of the law regarding death and dying. He discusses the law as it relates to both competent patients and those who are no longer able to make decisions for themselves. Increasingly, the law has recognized the right of competent individuals to reject medical treatment or intervention, even when such rejection will result in death. In discussing the scope of this right, Cantor examines such issues as forced nutrition and hydration, terminal sedation (or what Rousseau and Jackson prefer to call "palliative sedation"), limitations on the treatments that patients can demand when those treatments would be medically futile, and physician-assisted suicide. In reviewing the law as it relates to those who can no longer make decisions, Cantor discusses the appointment of a healthcare agent or proxy, advance medical directives, the "best interest of the patient" standard and what he calls the "constructive preference" standard that is sometimes invoked when the wishes of the patient have not been made clear in advance. The references at the end of this essay provide considerable guidance for those interested in pursuing legal issues related to death and dying.

It is now a truism to say that as medical technology advances, difficult decisions related to end-of-life issues multiply. The appropriate response is to recognize this and to do the preparatory thinking that will contribute to wisdom in such decision making. Toward that end this collection of essays is dedicated.

NOTES

Some of the ideas in this introduction are developed in more detail in Robert M. Baird, "Existentialism, Death, and Caring," *Journal of Religion and Health* 15, no. 2 (1976).

1. Martin Heidegger, *Being and Time* (New York: Harper and Row, 1962), p. 297.

2. Leo Tolstoy, *The Death of Ivan Ilych and Other Stories* (New York: New American Library, 1960), pp. 96–97.

3. Ibid., p. 99.

4. Ibid., p. 102.

5. Ibid., p. 103.

6. Ibid., pp. 131–32.

7. Jean-Paul Sartre, "The Wall," in *Existentialism from Dostoevsky to Sartre*, ed. Walter Kaufmann (Cleveland: Meridian Books, 1956), p. 227.

8. Ibid., p. 232.

9. Ibid., p. 233.

10. Ibid., pp. 234–35.

11. Tolstoy, *The Death of Ivan Ilych*, pp. 122–23.

12. Ibid., p. 125.

13. Ibid., p. 127.

14. Ibid., p. 131.

15. Paul Tillich, *The Courage to Be* (New Haven, Conn.: Yale University Press, 1952), p. 35.

16. Ibid., p. 45.

17. Ibid., p. 35.

18. Ibid., p.38.
19. Tolstoy, *The Death of Ivan Ilych*, pp. 129–30.
20. Ibid., p. 154.
21. Tillich, *The Courage to Be*, p. 86.
22. Ibid., p. 34.
23. Tolstoy, *The Death of Ivan Ilych*, pp. 155–56.
24. It should be noted that a volume devoted to euthanasia was previously published in the Contemporary Issues Series. Since that volume is soon to be updated and published in a revised version, the current collection of essays considers that issue only marginally. The question of assisted suicide is very much in the background of many of these essays, however.
25. This is the case in Oregon as a result of the 1997 Oregon Death with Dignity Act.

Part One

THE HOSPICE MOVEMENT

1

DEBUNKING THE MYTHS OF HOSPICE

Naomi Naierman

WHAT HOSPICE MEANS

Having access to hospice and the Medicare Hospice Benefit means that comprehensive care at the end of life does not have to be expensive or burdensome. Hospice means that we can die in comfort and dignity in our own home, with the support of and under the supervision of a coordinated team of professional staff and volunteers. Family members, too, will be supported in their caregiving roles and in their grief.

Hospice is a set of services that we all may need someday—if not for ourselves, then for our parents. Although death is not an option for any of us, we do have choices about the services we use at the end of life. Hospice is undoubtedly one of the best options in the last months of life because it offers a variety of benefits, not only to those of us who are dying, but also to those we leave behind.

Reprinted from *Choices: The Newsletter of Choice in Dying* 7, no. 3 (fall 1998), by permission of Partnership for Caring, 1620 Eye Street, NW, Suite 202, Washington, D.C. 20006 (800) 989–9455.

Yet, despite its many advantages, hospice is still a mystery to most Americans, even twenty-five years after its introduction in this country. That hospice remains a mystery is due in part to our society's resistance to discussing matters related to death. Also responsible is the federal government's poor performance in educating the public about the Medicare hospice program instituted in 1983. In addition, it is fair to say that, as a whole, hospices have not been effective in raising public awareness, either.

Now, more than ever, there is a sense of urgency to dispel the myths and to learn as much as possible about hospice. Otherwise, we will participate, albeit inadvertently, in the erosion of hospice and its benefits. The threats to hospice are undeniable, and they come from many directions. Among those threats is the reluctance of policymakers to use the word *hospice*, relying instead on words such as *palliation* or *palliative care*. As a result, even before hospice becomes a commonly understood concept, it could well disappear from our language.

Hospice programs throughout the country are facing a decrease in use of services due to government constraints. The federal government restricts hospice care to those whose death is six months away or sooner. Although the timing of death is difficult to predict, hospices are held accountable for accepting patients who outlive their six-month prognosis. Physicians, who in general refer patients to hospice only reluctantly, are increasingly more wary of government oversight of their prognostic decisions and their pain management practices. As a result, people who qualify for hospice care are referred too late, or not at all.

Managed care organizations (MCOs) may also create barriers to hospice. Most MCOs do not have financially rewarding arrangements with hospices; consequently, referring patients may mean financial losses, whereas using the MCO's own home health services may be financially more attractive. This situation constitutes a biased incentive that may not be favorable to dying patients.

Another threat to hospice is physician-assisted suicide, which could be all too readily substituted for hospice care, especially if dying people are not offered the hospice alternative in a timely way. Without the pain relief, emotional support, and spiritual guidance that hospice offers, physician-assisted suicide may look like a reasonable alternative to dying people in distress.

Ultimately, however, a public that is clueless about hospice is the most serious threat to the long-term survival of hospice in America. If we are not fully aware of the many benefits of hospice, we become prey to the vagaries of the healthcare system. On the other hand, if we are informed about the hospice concept, its comprehensive services, and its financial aspects, we can more fully participate in the decisions that doctors and policymakers are making on our behalf. If we learn about hospice, we can work to preserve it for the time that we, or someone we love, may need it.

COMMON MYTHS OF HOSPICE

To learn about hospice, it is useful to start by debunking the common myths that in themselves create barriers to hospice.[1]

MYTH #1. HOSPICE IS A PLACE.

Hospice care takes place wherever the need exists—usually the patient's home. About 80 percent of hospice care takes place in the home.

MYTH #2. HOSPICE IS *ONLY* FOR PEOPLE WITH CANCER.

More than one-fifth of hospice patients nationwide have diagnoses other than cancer. In urban areas, hospices serve a large number of HIV/AIDS patients. Increasingly, hospices are also serving families coping with the end stages of chronic diseases, such as emphysema, Alzheimer's, cardiovascular, and neuromuscular diseases.

MYTH #3. HOSPICE IS *ONLY* FOR OLD PEOPLE.

Although the majority of hospice patients are older, hospices serve patients of all ages. Many hospices offer clinical staff with expertise in pediatric hospice care.

MYTH #4. HOSPICE IS *ONLY* FOR DYING PEOPLE.

As a family-centered concept of care, hospice focuses as much on the grieving family as on the dying patients. Most hospices make their grief services available to the community at large, serving schools, churches, and the workplace.

MYTH #5. HOSPICE CAN HELP *ONLY* WHEN FAMILY MEMBERS ARE AVAILABLE TO PROVIDE CARE.

Recognizing that terminally ill people may live alone or with family members unable to provide care, many hospices coordinate community resources to make home care possible. Or they help to find an alternative location where the patient can safely receive care.

MYTH #6. HOSPICE IS FOR PEOPLE WHO DON'T NEED A HIGH LEVEL OF CARE.

Hospice is serious medicine. Most hospices are Medicare-certified, requiring that they employ experienced medical and nursing personnel with skills in symptom control. Hospices offer state-of-the-art palliative care, using advanced technologies to prevent or alleviate distressing symptoms.

MYTH #7. HOSPICE IS *ONLY* FOR PEOPLE WHO CAN ACCEPT DEATH.

While those affected by terminal illness struggle to come to terms with death, hospices gently help them find their way at their own speed. Many hospices welcome inquiries from families who are unsure about their needs and preferences. Hospice staff are readily available to discuss all options and to facilitate family decisions.

MYTH #8. HOSPICE CARE IS EXPENSIVE.

Most people who use hospice are over sixty-five and are entitled to the Medicare Hospice Benefit. This benefit covers virtually all hospice services and requires few, if any, out-of-pocket expenditures. This coverage reduces the family's financial burdens, and hospice care can be far less expensive than other end-of-life care.

MYTH #9. HOSPICE IS NOT COVERED BY MANAGED CARE.

Although managed care organizations (MCOs) are not required to include hospice coverage, Medicare beneficiaries can use their Medicare Hospice Benefit anytime, anywhere they choose. They are not locked into end-of-life services offered or not offered by the MCOs. On the other hand, those under sixty-five are confined to the MCO's services, but are likely to gain access to hospice care upon inquiry.

MYTH #10. HOSPICE IS FOR WHEN THERE IS NO HOPE.

When death is in sight, there are two options: submit without hope or live life as fully as ever until the end. The gift of hospice is its capacity to help families see how much can be shared at the end of life through personal and spiritual connections that often are not made otherwise. It is no wonder that many family members can look back upon their hospice experience with gratitude, and with the knowledge that everything possible was done toward a peaceful death.

WHAT IS HOSPICE?

Hospice includes medical care with an emphasis on pain management and symptom relief. Hospice teams of professionals and volunteers also address the emotional, social, and spiritual needs of the patient and the whole family. Overseeing all patient care is the hospice medical director who may also serve as the attending physician. Alternatively, the patient's own physician may continue in this role, in coordination with the hospice team and its plan of care.

MEDICAL CARE

Pain management is of particular concern for a patient with a life-threatening illness. Hospice staff are the experts in state-of-the-art pain treatments, helping patients feel comfortable with pain management alternatives. If administering pain medication at home requires a new skill, family members can count on the hospice staff for training and guidance.

Most medical treatment needed to make a terminally ill patient physically comfortable can be provided at home. Recent technological advances allow for a wide variety of equipment to be installed in the home, thus reducing the need for hospitalization, except in the most complicated cases. In rare cases when symptoms cannot be controlled at home, inpatient facilities are available.

EMOTIONAL AND SPIRITUAL SUPPORT

The fear of death can be due to the fear of pain and abandonment. Hospice staff include bereavement and spiritual counselors who help patients and families come to terms with dying. They assist patients in finishing important tasks, saying their final good-byes, healing broken family relationships, distributing precious objects, and completing a spiritual journey.

Unfinished business can make dying harder and grieving more difficult for those left behind. Hospice staff recognize that a person who comes to terms with dying has a less stressful death, and that the family benefits from a less complicated grieving process. A source of relief and comfort for many hospice patients is the knowledge that the family will receive ongoing bereavement support.

PRACTICAL CONSIDERATIONS

The day-to-day chores of life can become overwhelming for family caregivers. Hospice staff can teach them to care for the dying person at home. Family members learn how to administer medications, operate equipment, and coordinate services. Volunteers are integral members of the hospice staff, providing companionship and assistance in household chores.

FINANCIAL CONCERNS

Financial worries can be a major burden for a patient facing a terminal illness. Most hospice patients are Medicare participants with ready access to a hospice benefit that minimizes out-of-pocket expenses in the last months of life. The Medicare Hospice Benefit covers prescribed medications, visits by medical and nursing professionals, home health aides, short-term inpatient care, and bereavement support for the family after the patient has died. The Medicare Hospice Benefit also eliminates the burden of paperwork, as families are not required to submit claims or pay bills. For patients without hospice insurance, financial accommodations are made based on the ability to pay.

HOSPICE: THE CHALLENGE TO AMERICAN HEALTHCARE CONSUMERS

Hospice as a concept suffers from a powerful denial syndrome in our society. Hospice must be better understood if it is to reach all who need it. When all Americans know what hospice is, they are more likely to make it an explicit part of their long-term plans, and their fear of death will be abated. Increased visibility of hospice locally and nationally will result in more people becoming active advocates for themselves and for their families.

WHAT LACK OF HOSPICE KNOWLEDGE CAN MEAN

If you don't know all about hospice, you may

- die in pain, especially if you are in a hospital or nursing home. Studies show that a majority of people who die in these institutions die in pain. People die in pain because hospital and nursing home staff often lack adequate skills in pain management. Hospice staff are the experts in pain management and can virtually guarantee a comfortable death.
- be sent home from the hospital with home health services that are not comprehensive and are not provided by staff trained in end-of-life care. For example, prescription drugs, which are not covered by Medicare under home healthcare, are especially costly.
- have difficulty getting hospice care if you live in a nursing home. You have a right to hospice care, regardless of where you live. And, if you are over sixty-five, you are entitled to a comprehensive hospice benefit.
- leave behind family, friends, and relatives without support

through their mourning period. Only hospice programs offer this support free of charge for at least a year after death.

NOTE

1. Adapted from Naomi Naierman and Jo A. Turner, "Demystifying Hospice," *AAPA News* (15 July 1997): 7.

2

A COMPARISON OF HOSPICE IN THE U.K. AND THE U.S.

Karen Y. Chapman and Lessie Bass

INTRODUCTION

The modern hospice movement is recognized as a direct result of the tireless work of Dr. Cicely Saunders, the founder of the United Kingdom's St. Christopher's Hospice in 1967.[1] Though the United States modeled its first hospice after St. Christopher's, there are differences between the two countries in their hospice programs. Most hospice services in the United States are provided in the patient's home, while just the opposite occurs in the United Kingdom, where most hospice services take place within the inpatient setting. According to Ann Eve, A. M. Smith, and Peter Tebbit, however, the trend in the U.K. over the last five years has been toward provision of services in the home.[2]

Much of the data for the United Kingdom was obtained in England during the summer of 1997 through study under the Bristol International Credit-Earning Programme (BICEP) at the Univer-

Reprinted from *American Journal of Hospice & Palliative Care* 17, no. 3 (May/June 2000): 173–77.

sity of Bristol. In addition, Ann Eve, information officer at the Hospice Information Service, and Peter Tebbit, National Palliative Care Development Advisor, were instrumental in finding information. It is our hope that this article will serve as a foundation resource for others who are completing research on comparisons of hospice care within the two countries.

Having had the opportunity to observe two hospices in the southwest region of the United Kingdom, in Bristol and Devon, we found that these—as well as most in the United Kingdom—largely rely on donations, grants, and volunteers to maintain their status, since they receive only a small portion of their funding from the National Health Service (NHS). Hospices in the United States also continue to rely upon solicited grants and donations as partial funding resources, with additional funds coming from insurance, under Medicare, Medicaid, private insurance companies, or the Veterans Administration.

BRIEF HISTORICAL DEVELOPMENT

UNITED KINGDOM

One of the earliest institutions in England to provide care to the dying was St. Joseph's Hospice.[3] It was established by the English Sisters of Charity in 1905 and was the place where Dr. Cicely Saunders "refined the ideas and protocols that formed the cornerstone of modern hospice care" during the 1950s and 1960s.[4]

In the United Kingdom, hospice care is categorized under "specialist palliative care services." This type of care integrates the physical, psychological, social, and spiritual aspects of care for the support of the patient and family during illness, periods of recovery, dying, and after the patient's death.[5]

UNITED STATES

In addition to being an influential figure in England, Dr. Saunders was a prominent person in the development of the hospice concept in the United States. In 1963 she spoke to a group of medical students at Yale University about her work,[6] and at that time met Florence Wald, who was the dean of nursing. Wald invited Dr. Saunders to return in 1966 to provide a hospice workshop[7] and she in turn visited St. Christopher's to observe and conduct research on establishing hospice services. Wald later was instrumental in the opening of the first hospice in the United States, in 1974 in Connecticut, offering home care and bereavement services.[8]

Dr. Elisabeth Kübler-Ross was a significant figure in the development of hospice in the United States. She increased public awareness of life, death, and the importance of the modern hospice movement. Her book *Death and Dying*[9] was based upon a series of interviews with dying patients. She identified the five stages of the dying process. Those five stages are also frequently used as a basis for discussing the grieving process.

The contributing works of Saunders, Wald, and Kübler-Ross, as well as the increasing acceptance by the public, assisted in the development of hospice in the United States. The final stage of life was finally being celebrated with dignity and respect.

FUNDING

UNITED KINGDOM

Provision of hospice services in the United Kingdom is not dependent upon a patient or family's ability to pay. Services are provided on a "no charge" basis to patients or their general practitioner (GP), who is the gatekeeper for accessing services. It is the GP who certifies that a patient's condition is terminal. The

National Association of Health Authorities and Trusts defines a terminal illness as an "active and progressive disease for which curative treatment is not possible or not appropriate and from which death can reasonably be expected within twelve months."[10]

Some hospices are totally funded and managed by the NHS while others rely heavily upon fund-raising activities and philanthropic donations. Hospices in the United Kingdom depend on a variety of resources to meet the medical needs of patients and their families. Contributions from the NHS are obtained through grants from trusts and health authorities.[11]

In addition to these contributions, the Cancer Relief MacMillan Fund provides initial funds (for the first three years) to many of the home nursing teams, after which the health authority assumes the responsibility for funding.[12] Other foundations, such as the Sue Ryder Foundation, provide funding for many hospice homes throughout the United Kingdom to help defray the cost of care. The Sue Ryder homes care for patients afflicted with a wide variety of diseases and disabilities in addition to providing palliative care services tailored to the needs of each patient and family.[13] The Marie Curie Nurses' Support and Marie Curie Cancer Care are examples of resources that are accessed through the health authorities.[14] Outpatient clinics provide palliative care services, and some privately owned nursing homes also offer care to the terminally ill.[15]

UNITED STATES

Prior to 1983, most hospices relied exclusively upon grants, private donations, and volunteers to meet the needs of patients and their families.[16]

Reimbursement through any insurance entity was not a reality at that time. Most eligible hospices currently can receive reimbursement from Medicare, Medicaid, the Veterans Administration, and private insurance companies. In addition, hospices do a great deal of their own fund-raising and also rely on donations.

The Medicare Hospice Benefit was introduced in 1983[17] and became a permanent part of Medicare coverage in 1986 for those eligible.[18] The benefit falls under Medicare Part A, which is hospital insurance. Almost 80 percent of hospices are Medicare-certified,[19] and patients must meet eligibility requirements. First, one's primary physician must certify that the person is terminally ill, meaning that person has a life expectancy of six months or less.[20] Second, the hospice must be Medicare-certified to receive reimbursement for services rendered to patients and their families. Third, treatment received must be for "management of a terminal illness."[21] Additional services, including duplication of services provided by another hospice or other providers, may be needed and rendered in order to provide a continuum of care, but will not be covered by Medicare.[22] There are four benefit periods. According to a 1995 National Hospice Organization (NHO) survey, 65.3 percent of patients were covered by the Medicare Hospice Benefit.[23]

In 1995, Medicaid covered about 12 percent of hospice patients.[24] The Medicaid Hospice Benefit program covers some expenses not included in the Medicare Hospice Benefit. Forty-one states and the District of Columbia accept this benefit. The program also offers each state the choice of excluding persons infected with acquired immune deficiency syndrome (AIDS).[25] Medicaid has four predetermined rates for each day of care.[26] These rates are dependent on the type of services that the patient received for the day, which may include inpatient care or routine home care.[27]

The Veterans Health Administration offers hospice services through some Veterans Administration (VA) medical centers. These centers hold the option of contracting for patient services with local hospices.[28]

Eighty-two percent of managed care plans offer hospice services and most private insurance companies currently reimburse for hospice services.[29] Managed care coverage varies from policy to policy; however, physician, nursing, medical social work, and certified nursing assistant services are usually reimbursed on a consistent "per-visit basis."[30]

In 1995, the Civilian Health and Medical Program of the Uniformed Services (CHAMPUS/TriCare) joined other organizations in the authorization of coverage for hospice care for patients and their families).[31]

REGULATORY STANDARDS

UNITED KINGDOM

Hospices in the United Kingdom operate under self-imposed regulations. Each hospice has its own set of criteria that varies.[32] According to the Working Party on Guidelines in Palliative Care:[33]

> There is talk of accreditation of hospices by outside bodies, but as yet there is no existing professional machinery to perform this duty.
> There also is no indication of universal acceptance that [accreditation] standards will be accepted in favor of the self-imposed arrangements.[34]

The United Kingdom National Council for Hospice and Specialist Palliative Care Service and the Hospice Information Service at St. Christopher's also provide research and resource information, as well as advocacy for the terminally ill.

UNITED STATES

There is no mandatory accrediting body in the United States. The Health Care Financing Administration (HCFA) serves as the regulatory body for Medicare-certified hospices and there are state licensures. There are also organizations that provide voluntary accreditation. The Joint Commission Accreditation of Healthcare

Organizations (JCAHO) and the National League for Nursing Community Health Accreditation Program (CHAP) are two accrediting bodies for hospices in the United States.[35] Regulatory procedures generally include the completion of on-site surveys, which focus on patient satisfaction and compliance with rules related to the provision of care, and the minimum acceptable practice level.[36]

The National Hospice and Palliative Care Organization (NHPCO, formerly NHO) is a nonprofit public benefit charitable organization, which advocates for the needs of the terminally ill in the United States.[37] Furthermore, this organization possesses a wealth of information on hospices throughout the country.

DEMOGRAPHICS

UNITED KINGDOM

At the time of this study, there were 125 independent voluntary inpatient hospices, eleven Marie Curie homes, and nine Sue Ryder Foundation homes in the United Kingdom.[38]

Inpatient Units

Eve et al.[39] surveyed providers of palliative care services. The survey included inpatient, home care, and day care providers. In 1994–1995, 30,063 new patients were admitted to palliative care units. There were slightly more females (50.3 percent) than males (49.7 percent). The average length of stay was 13.5 days. Fifty-four percent of deaths occurred at the unit.

Table 1 shows that the predominant ethnic group was white (98.4 percent). Cancer was the major disease among this population, and 65 percent of the population were over sixty-five years old.[40]

Table 1. Ethnicity and Diagnosis of Inpatient Clients

Ethnicity

98.4% white
0.7% black (includes African, Caribbean, and other)
0.5% Indian, Pakistani, and Bengali
0.1% Chinese
0.3% other

Diagnosis

96.7% cancer
1.3% neurological
0.5% HIV/AIDS
0.4% cardiovascular
1.2% other

Source: A. Eve, A. M. Smith, P. Tebbit, "Hospice and Palliative Care in the U.K. 1994–1995," *Palliative Medicine* 11 (1997): 31–43.

Home Care

The home care population showed similar results. There were 40,375 new patients admitted. Sixty percent of the patients were over sixty-five years old, with 51.4 percent female and 48.6 percent male. Some 96.3 percent of the patients had cancer. The average length of stay was two to three months, with the largest number (46 percent) dying at home, 26 percent in a palliative care unit, 23 percent in a hospital, and 5 percent in a nursing home.[41]

UNITED STATES

At the time of this study, there were approximately three thousand operational or planned hospices in the fifty states, the District of Columbia, and Puerto Rico.[42] According to a 1994–1995 survey completed by NHO, 450,000 patients were helped by hospice.[43]

Table 2. Demographics in the United States

Provision of services	Gender	Age	Ethnicity	Diagnosis	Average length of stay	Place of death
90% at home	52% male 48% female	71% of males > 65 years old 74% of females > 65 years old	83% white 8% African American 3% Hispanic 6% other	60% cancer 6% heart diagnosis 3% AIDS 2% Alzheimer's 1% renal failure 2% other	61.5 days	77% personal residence 19% institutional facility 4% other

Source: NHO Fact Sheet, 1997.

Table 2 shows the demographics of the population. Ninety percent of hospice services were delivered in the home, the percentage of males was higher than that of females, and the majority of the patients were over sixty-five years old. Cancer was the major diagnosis, and whites were the predominant group to receive services.[44]

CONCLUSION

There are some similarities between hospice in the United States and in the United Kingdom. Dr. Cicely Saunders played an instrumental role in the establishment of the modern hospice movement in both countries. Hospices in both countries rely on a variety of funding sources. In each country the primary physician serves as the gatekeeper to services. The philosophy of hospice remains the same. Volunteers are a major support system in both countries.

There is no mandatory accreditation in either country. There are voluntary accrediting organizations in the United States. Hospices in the United Kingdom rely on self-imposed standards. However, the JCAHO is preparing new guidelines for hospice and home care accreditation, with these scheduled to go into effect in 2001.

The majority of services in the United States are provided at home. As previously noted, hospice at home is becoming a trend in the United Kingdom. Cancer is the major diagnosis in both countries. The majority of the population is white with many patients over sixty-five years of age.

Some of the data in this article is at least two years old, allowing additional updated demographic information to be collected in future research studies.

NOTES

1. G. Ford, "A palliative care system: The Marie Curie model," *Am J Hosp Palliat Care* (1993): 27.

2. A. Eve, A. M. Smith, and P. Tebbit, "Hospice and palliative care in the U.K. 1994–95," *Palliat Med* 11 (1997): 31–43. Includes a summary of trends, 1990–95.

3. H. Taylor, *The Hospice Movement in Britain: Its Role and Its Future* (London: Center for Policy on Aging, 1983).

4. M. O. Amentia, "The hospice movement," in *Nursing Care of the Terminally Ill*, ed. M. O. Amentia and N. L. Bohnet (Boston: Little, Brown and Co., 1986), p. 53.

5. Working Party on Clinical Guidelines in Palliative Care, *Information for Purchasers: Background to Available Specialist Palliative Care Services*, drafted by Dr. Gillian Ford (London: National Council for Hospice and Specialist Palliative Care Services, 1995).

6. D. A. Bennahum, "The historical development of hospice and palliative care," in *Hospice and Palliative Care: Concepts and Practice*, ed. D. C. Sheehan and W. B. Forman (Sudbury, Mass.: Jones and Bartlett, 1996).

7. Ibid.

8. Ibid.

9. E. Kübler-Ross, *On Death and Dying* (New York: Macmillian, 1969).

10. NHS executive letter, 23 February 1995. Annex A.

11. M. Robbins, P. Jackson, and A. Prentice, *Palliative Cancer Provision in the Southwest* (Bristol, U.K.: University of Bristol, 1994).

12. T. Jones, *The Structure of the National Health Service* (Beckenham, Kent, U.K.: Publishing Initiatives, 1997).

13. Sue Ryder Foundation, "The founders," [online], www.employees.org/~anand/ raphael/leosue.html [5 April 1998].

14. Jones, *The Structure of the National Health Service.*

15. Ibid.

16. J. Rhymes, "Hospice in America," *JAMA* 264, no. 3 (1990): 369.

17. Ibid.

18. J. E. Neigh, "History of hospice in the United States," *Caring* 12 (1993): 11.

19. National Hospice Organization (NHO), "NHO hospice fact sheet," (1997): 1–2.

20. National Hospice Organization, "Medicare Hospice Benefit," [online], www.nho.org/medicare/htm [5 August 1997].

21. Ibid.

22. Ibid.

23. Ibid.

24. NHO, "Hospice fact sheet," pp. 1–2.

25. Health Care Financing Administration (HCFA), "Hospice services," [online], www.hcfa.gov/medicaid/ltc2.htm [9 September 1997].

26. NHO, "Hospice fact sheet," pp. 1–2.

27. HCFA, "Hospice services."

28. J. Vermilion, "The referral process and reimbursement," in *Hospice and Palliative Care: Concepts and Practice,* ed. D. C Sheehan and W. B. Forman (Sudbury, Mass.: Jones and Bartlett, 1996).

29. NHO, "Hospice fact sheet," pp. 1–2.

30. Vermilion, "Referral process."

31. NHO, "Hospice fact sheet," pp. 1–2.

32. A. Eve and P. Tebbit, personal communication, August 1997.

33. Working Party on Clinical Guidelines in Palliative Care, "Information for purchasers."

34. Ibid., p. 16.

35. B. L. Schmoll and C. E. Dixon, "Quality care in hospice," in *Hospice and Palliative Care: Concepts and Practice,* ed. D. C. Sheehan and W. B. Forman (Sudbury, Mass.: Jones and Bartlett, 1996).

36. Ibid.

37. NHO, "Hospice fact sheet," pp. 1–2.

38. Jones, *The Structure of the National Health Service.*

39. Eve, Smith, and Tebbit, "Hospice and palliative care in the U.K. 1994–95," pp. 31–43.

40. Ibid.

41. Ibid.

42. NHO, "Hospice fact sheet," pp. 1–2.

43. Ibid.

44. Ibid.

3

CHANGING THE GAME IN THE INTENSIVE CARE UNIT
Letting Nature Take Its Course

Helen S. Chapple

It sounds simple enough: "We've done everything we could to save him, and it hasn't worked. Now it's time to withdraw aggressive treatment, maintain comfort, and let Nature take its course." So patients' families and clinicians may describe the decision to withdraw life support. The phrase, "letting Nature take its course" has an appeal. The concept seems to represent a return to wholeness, to simple existence and process, something different from the assault of catheters and infusions and noisy machines. We like the restful sound of it.

In reality, death in the intensive care unit (ICU) is neither simple nor natural. We would like to see things happen "naturally," but our interferences in Nature's course up to the point of making the decision to withdraw life support have eliminated this possibility. The healthcare team is responsible for imposing the complex interventions that stabilized the patient's condition, and we cannot just turn everything off and walk away. (For the purposes of this discussion, the withdrawal of life support includes discontinuing any intervention that might have necessitated admission to the ICU, such as mechanical ventilation, administration of vasopressors, and the need for intensive monitoring.) We need to manage the approach of death with the same skill, sophistication, and compassion that characterized the interventions we used to keep the patient alive so far, and in an ideal world, we would do just that. Dying would look as seamless and as whole as we imagine Nature to be. The problem is that terminal care is the precipice where our ICU knowledge and sophistication ends. Death is not the mission of any ICU, and we do not know how to manage dying.

TERMINAL CARE AS A GAME

To understand the magnitude of the problem, we can compare terminal care to a game with which we are unfamiliar. Before the rules and strategies of any game make sense to us, we need to know the endpoint that we are after, the object of the game. Rescuing a patient whose condition is unstable is a serious game that we are quite comfortable playing in the ICU. The object is clear: saving the patient's life. The rules and strategies of cardiopulmonary resuscitation (i.e., airway, breathing, circulation) and Advanced Cardiac Life Support algorithms, constantly refined and updated, tell us how to play the game with the best chance of success.

Withdrawing life support occurs at the other end of the ICU spectrum, and we may engage in this care more often than we treat emergent unstable conditions in our patients. Yet, unlike the clarity and crispness of the guidelines that govern rescue, no universally accepted rules or standards of care exist to guide our practices in terminal care. Furthermore, no mechanisms are in place to measure the quality of care we deliver to patients at the end of life.[1]

The conscious initiation and subsequent management of a patient's dying process are often the responsibilities of nurses. Physicians, ethicists, and others may play an active role in the decision making that precedes the withdrawal of life support, but after the decision is made, the ethicists leave and the physicians may wish to shift their focus to the "still viable" patients, leaving the care of the dying patient to the nurses and the respiratory therapist.[2] It is often up to a nurse to shift a life-prolonging care plan 180 degrees to include the expected death of the patient. The nurse who manages these details becomes the "referee" and the "coach" for the new game of terminal care (see case report 1).

Without a clear understanding of the object of the game or its rules, patients' care at the end of life is subject to dangerous inconsistency. The healthcare team may organize care according to whatever goal seems important to team members. If the object of the game in terminal care were patients' comfort, the rules might indeed mandate unlimited use of pain medication given as needed, even though this practice creates a conflict for nurses.[3] Little oversight or accountability would be needed for bedside practice, so long as the patient's comfort was maintained. Or, suppose the object of the game were to minimize the disruption of the care being delivered to other patients in the unit. In that case, other rules might apply, such as providing support for the family of the dying patient and for staff members in the hope that no one would make a scene, transferring the patient to the ward or hospice unit as soon as possible, maintaining a professional (unemotional) demeanor, and giving the patient medications as needed to preserve the atmosphere of calm.

In fact, no object of the game of terminal care has been specified, and clear ethical problems are associated with using comfort or peace as the true measure of excellence in care delivery at the end of life. Drawing a bright, clear line between comfort care and euthanasia is difficult for both clinicians in practice and bioethicists.[4] Death is often a messy and complicated business. The dying process can be distasteful and indeed abhorrent to ICU clinicians, who specialize in creating order out of chaos, rather than the other way around. If no death can be a good death in the ICU, dying patients can at least be well medicated, which is to say death can be hastened in the interest of comfort or peace,[5] the root meaning of the word "euthanasia."

THE SEARCH FOR A GOOD DEATH

Still, a good death may have a broader meaning than simply the patient's comfort or peace. A good death that did not mean euthanasia, still illegal in all states, might even be a worthy object of the game of ICU terminal care. Several studies[6] help us understand what a good death is not (prolonged aggressive treatment, no communication, no choices, too much pain).

The literature and the Internet present several approaches to defining the goals of terminal care when life support is withdrawn. We find treatment of death and dying from the bioethics perspective, prescriptions by acute care experts, guidelines from professional organizations, and discussions of specific clinical issues:

- Bioethics in death and dying traditionally concerns itself with the ethics of the decision-making process, the definition of death, the validity of treatment refusal, physician-assisted suicide, and considerations about giving pain medication that is thought to shorten the patient's life.[7]
- Prescriptions for excellent terminal care when life support is withdrawn emphasize comfort, dignity (which is difficult to define, especially from the perspective of the dying patient),[8] patient- and family-centered choice, and communication.[9]
- The American Medical Association[10] and Last Acts[11] have issued guidelines for end-of-life care generally and for the

withdrawal of intensive care specifically. The Society for Critical Care Medicine and the American Thoracic Society have also issued guidelines, but those guidelines[12] address the difficulties in decision making at the end of life rather than the implementation of the decision. The position of the American Nurses Association on the nurse's role emphasizes refraining from participation in physician-assisted suicide and euthanasia and encouraging patients' choices.[13] Although these statements are helpful in a general way, they define neither the parameters of a good outcome nor the strategies that clinicians might use to bring about a good outcome.

🍂 Articles about particular practice issues and the ethical implications of the issues when life support is withdrawn include topics such as terminal weaning from mechanical ventilation versus extubation,[14] use of neuromuscular blockade,[15] and controversial use of medications.[16] These discussions familiarize us with important pieces of the puzzle, but they do not show us the picture on the outside of the box.

Although the literature does not satisfy us by defining a goal for our terminal care, or by sketching the outlines of what constitutes a good death after the withdrawal of life support, it does suggest a multifaceted ideal for terminal care aimed at expanding the universe of choices available to patients and their families when death becomes an expected part of the care plan. Unfortunately, in practice, the decision to withdraw life support often telescopes this complexity into the phrase *comfort care only*.

In addition, another wrinkle exists. Without an object of the game, we cannot know when we have "won." Without outcome standards or models of excellence tailored to the withdrawal of life support, we cannot measure the quality of terminal care. Ethical and professional standards regarding the decision-making process are clear, but we cannot evaluate our hands-on management of a patient's dying process. The standards of the Joint Commission on Accreditation of Healthcare Organizations[17] for end-of-life care are not specific enough to be helpful. Terminal care after the withdrawal of life support may be more devoid of regulation and oversight than any other nursing or medical practice. This situation is especially ironic when we consider the attention that we pay to the ethics of the decision making that precedes withdrawal of life support.

HOSPICE CARE AND A GOOD DEATH

Although neither the literature nor professional standards describe what constitutes a good death after the withdrawal of life support, some clinicians have explored the concept of a good death in theory and in practice. Hospices' terminal care experts assume that the dying process itself contains an ethical good. (Ellen McGee[18] contends that this underlying assumption of good in the dying process is what makes suicidal ideation so problematic for hospices.) That ethical good can be obtained by the participants merely by paying attention. When the object of the game is paying attention to the dying process, the rules and strategies for playing the game follow logically: namely, life is not prolonged, and dying is not hastened; the patient and the patient's family make up the unit of care, and they define what works best for them; and multidisciplinary attention is paid to controlling troublesome symptoms and to the patient's spiritual, psychological, and social needs (see table 1).

The reputation of hospice care for palliation of symptoms is well known. What is less obvious is the fact that expert control of symptoms is a means to an end for hospice care. Hospice clinicians and volunteers want to solve problems and remove distractions that stand in the way of achieving the good that can be found in the dying process. The nature of that good is presumably variable

Table 1 Comparison of Terminal Care Settings

Rules of the game in hospice care	Goals for terminal care in the intensive care unit
1. Life is not prolonged, and death is not hastened.	1. Patient's comfort and safety.
2. Comfort is a means to an end.	2. Opportunity to honor the patient's life and mark the significance of its end.
3. The patient and the patient's family form the unit of care.	3. No abandonment.
4. Multidisciplinary attention is paid to control of signs and symptoms and to spiritual, psychological, and social needs.	4. Moral stability for all participants.
	5. Support for the patient and the patient's family, including choice, communication, and participation.

and subject to personal definition by the participants, but the good can include enjoying the time that is left, preparing for the death, and finding whatever meaning might be available in the situation. Participants and caregivers often attest to a richness about the dying experience with hospice support. Hospice care plays its game of terminal care on a playing field that is conducive to enhancing the meaning of such a profound experience: the home of the patient.

Hospice care was invented because hospitals were not good at the game of terminal care. Over the years, hospice personnel have used the home setting to hone their skills and develop the game of hospice care to a high level of refinement with a unique set of rules and a pace all its own. Extending the analogy, we can think of hospice care as something similar to the game of baseball played on a baseball diamond, a field well suited to the game's goals. Play unfolds at its own pace, a single batter at a time, with each batter claiming the total attention of the field as he/she steps up to the plate.

By contrast, healthcare delivered in the ICU resembles the game of football: aggressive, relentless, fast paced, highly stimulating. When we deliver terminal care to a dying patient in the ICU, we are attempting to play baseball on the gridiron while the football game is in full swing. A top priority is to avoid being trampled.

Attention is the most fundamental requirement for playing any

---

CASE REPORT 1

A twenty-year-old man, Mr. M, is a patient in the neurological intensive care unit with a gunshot wound to the head. He breathes on his own but satisfies other neurological criteria for death. Mr. M's family has decided not to donate organs and wants life support to be withdrawn. All family members have gone home, expecting to be called when Mr. M dies. Mr. M is in the unit's only double room, and his roommate is watching television. The unit is full, and a patient with a cervical spinal cord injury is waiting in the emergency department for a space to become available in the unit. The plan is to extubate Mr. M and transfer him to the general ward as soon as his condition is stable, making a place for the new patient. After extubation, Mr. M has airway obstruction. The noise he makes with each breath is audible to the entire unit and very disconcerting. A manual jaw thrust eliminates the noise. While the nurses and the respiratory therapist discuss what to do, they take turns holding Mr. M's jaw in place to keep his respirations quiet. The unit has a draft protocol to help staff members manage the withdrawal of life support, but neither administering the recommended doses of 1 to 2 mg of morphine nor repositioning Mr. M have solved the problem. The house officer has ducked her head in to check on things but has not intervened. The respiratory therapist advocates giving Mr. M enough morphine to knock out the respiratory drive in the interest of the patient's comfort. One nurse rejects this plan as euthanasia, and the other nurse does not have a strong opinion. Per the suggestion of the second nurse, a slightly higher dose of a 4 mg intravenous bolus of morphine

---

game, especially when the game is unfamiliar. When we withdraw life support, we must leave the customary ICU routine, focus on a game for which the rules and the skills are unspecified, and play

is given, but nothing changes. At the insistence of the first nurse, the respiratory therapist inserts an oral airway. The patient exhibits no distress, the noise ceases, and the patient is transferred to the general ward.

Case discussion: The patient waiting in the emergency department, the noise of Mr. M's breathing, and Mr. M's alert roommate exerted silent pressure on the clinicians to move rapidly. The absence of Mr. M's family gave them the freedom to work among themselves. The oral airway might have been the first intervention, but the respiratory therapist hesitated to use it for fear it would cause the patient discomfort. The respiratory therapist also saw no benefit in allowing this devastated patient to continue to live. The respiratory therapist said that should he ever be in a similar situation, "I hope no one stands around my bedside talking about me."

When the guidelines provided by the protocol were insufficient, the clinicians negotiated the plan among themselves on the basis of their own experiences and personal biases. The only values articulated among them were the patient's comfort and avoiding euthanasia, and these values competed for ascendancy. The unspoken goals were not really the comfort of the patient (he appeared unaffected by these changes), but rather comfort and calm for the team, the rest of the unit, and the ward receiving the patient. Speed of transfer was also a priority because of the pending admission. No guidance or oversight was provided by the physician (although the physician could have done so), and no terminal care documentation form was available (as there would have been for a code) for documenting the events or the negotiation that occurred.

the game on a field that is unfriendly. In this situation, it may seem easier to behave as though baseball is really just a variation of football.

CASE REPORT 2

Seventy-eight-year-old Miss B came to the unit five weeks ago because of complications from Parkinson's disease. She had seizures soon after admission, and her condition deteriorated because of unknown causes. She had been minimally responsive during the past few weeks. Most of the nurses had cared for her at some point and knew that her sister was unrealistic about the prognosis. In the past two days, Miss B's kidneys had failed, and another family meeting was held. Miss B's sister agreed to the withdrawal of life support and then left the hospital, because the death "might not come for six hours." She expected to return after the death. The unit was full, and this patient was part of a two-patient assignment for the charge nurse during a twelve-hour day shift. The process of withdrawal began at 6:30 P.M., thirty minutes before change of shift at 7 P.M. Shortly before 7 P.M., a nurse and a respiratory therapist who were coming on for the night shift found themselves at the patient's bedside. They wondered if it was appropriate to remove the ventilator from her tracheostomy (the normal practice on the unit) or to leave the ventilator attached and reduce oxygen support over time. Miss B was too weak to draw a breath that would "trigger the vent," indicating that she could move no air into her lungs at all. The therapist argued that to

Case Report 2 illustrates the distress that can occur when clinicians are not comfortable with the plan for terminal care. It shows how ICU routines can steamroll and flatten the process of dying. Clinicians sense an almost overwhelming pressure when the workload is heavy to "keep going," to get on with whatever comes next and get the job done.[19] Often it is not easy to stop, think about what is different about death, and approach terminal care for the patient in a more appropriate way.

take away all support was active euthanasia. The hubbub of shift change ended the discussion, and their questions never reached the charge nurse. The night nurse began the receiving report on her assignment while the charge nurse obtained 4 mg of morphine from the lockbox. When the night nurse realized at 7:20 P.M. that the process of withdrawal had to be interrupted, Miss B had already died. The nurse started to cry and said, "This didn't need to be rushed. We've had this patient for weeks. We didn't have to withdraw at change of shift." Hearing this statement, the charge nurse exploded, said she would not be accused of disrespect, and abruptly left the unit.

Case discussion: Miss B's situation includes some features similar to those in Mr. M's case: absence of family, lack of involvement of physicians, and the need for negotiation. Miss B's respiratory compromise was more profound than usually seen in neurology patients. The benefits and burdens of departing from customary unit practice to accommodate her condition would have taken some time to discuss. Miss B may or may not have benefited from the ensuing delay. But because the withdrawal process began so close to shift change, clinicians with moral standing in her care could not share her final moments or have significant input in how her signs and symptoms might be managed.

GOALS FOR TERMINAL CARE IN THE ICU

A decision to withdraw life support, ethically made, does not often address the hands-on management issues that surround the dying process. Without a shared understanding of outcomes and standards, chaotic care can result. Hospice personnel have such a shared understanding of the terminal care they provide, but the context of hospice practice and the longer death trajectory of hospice patients makes translation of that understanding into ICU practice problematic.

A good death in the hospice sense is not an unreasonable object of the game for terminal care in the ICU. Ethical goals are relevant even when death may come in minutes or hours, rather than in days or weeks, as is usually the case in hospice care.

When we are able to separate our terminal care from the ICU routine and attend to our patient's dying process, comfort for the patient and support for the patient's family are usually our primary concerns. With the time and the energy to reflect on other important moral goals, we would want to ensure the following (see table 1):

- We want to honor the patient's life and mark the significance of its end. This is the only time that this patient is ever going to die.
- We do not want to abandon the patient or the patient's family. In fact, we want to invite their participation in these final decisions. We should include disclosure about the process, offer choices, and encourage patients and their families to be a part of the care, according to their desires and comfort levels.
- We all need a sense of moral stability. No one should be wondering after the death whether he/she or someone else may have killed the patient.
- We must ensure patients' safety and their right to take their own time to die. As long as patients are comfortable, their dying must be allowed to unfold in whatever way that it will. (Only if the patient has neuromuscular blocking agents in his or her system that cannot be reversed should high doses of sedatives and opioids be administered on a presumptive basis.)

We can adopt a vision of terminal care that regards comfort as a means to an end, and that end can be a good death, similar to the hospice concept. But when we must play baseball on a football field, the hospice game of terminal care must be altered substantially to account for the demands of our football context. Most football players are not cross-trained to play baseball. Similarly, many critical care clinicians have neither the time nor the desire to explore death education principles or hospice training. Although a proposal to attach hospicelike units next to the ICU would carve out a handy nearby baseball field to receive these patients,[20] this practice is not a near-term solution for most critical care clinicians.

Between the decision to withdraw life support and the actual death of the patient is an important period. We can divide this period into two segments: the time between the decision to withdraw life support and the clinical implementation of that decision and the time between the actual withdrawal and the patient's death (see figure 1). In the following sections, these periods are examined in reverse chronological order, starting with the period after withdrawal of life support, when the patient is actively dying.

BETWEEN THE WITHDRAWAL OF LIFE SUPPORT AND THE DEATH: ATTENDING TO THE DYING PROCESS

Acute care clinicians are accustomed to memory devices and acronyms (ABCs for airway, breathing, circulation; "look, listen, and feel"; and RACE for rescue, alarm, contain, extinguish [in response to a fire]) that we use to remind us of key strategies in stressful situations. When we withdraw life support, we need a simple statement to acknowledge the fact that a new game has started on our inhospitable field and to orient us to our new priorities of care: *Dying is a process, and attending to the dying process is an ethical end in itself.* Attending to the dying process means recognizing that an important course of events has been set in motion and that we must organize our care to pay attention to its effects.

Figure 1. Period between the Decision to Withdraw Life Support and the Implementation of That Decision

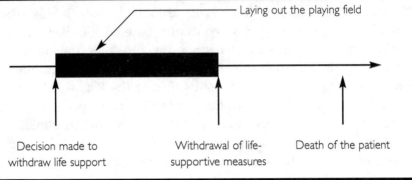

Laying out the playing field

Decision made to withdraw life support

Withdrawal of life-supportive measures

Death of the patient

DYING IS A PROCESS

The first half of the statement, *dying is a process*, acknowledges that some amount of time exists (minutes, hours, or days) between the moment that we withdraw life support and the moment the patient's heart stops beating. During this interval, the patient's physical condition will undoubtedly change. Some of these changes are predictable (breathing pattern, blood pressure, heart rate, and skin color), and some are not (level of the patient's discomfort, reactions of the patient's family, length of time). These changes have significance for caregivers and for the patient's family as we observe the approach of death, and this period can be used to adjust and respond to these changes. We are on slippery ethical ground if we do not acknowledge that dying is a process and allow it to unfold in its own way.

ATTENDING TO THE DYING PROCESS IS AN ETHICAL END IN ITSELF

The second half of the statement, *attending to the dying process is an ethical end in itself*, points out the need for "solidarity in mortality."[21] We acknowledge our ultimate lack of control in the face of death. As critical care clinicians, we are accustomed to a fair amount of authority over the body systems of our patients. The prospect of allowing anything about our patient to "unfold in its own way" can make us extremely uncomfortable. Our obligation to the patient and the patient's family during the dying process is not to look away, but to attend to the changes we see happening. First, our attention ensures the patient's comfort. The patient's physiological changes will require adjustments in our interventions with positioning, pain medication, and explanations and reassurance for the patient's family. Second, our attention to the dying process facilitates our accomplishment of the ethical goals of honoring the death, providing support, and ensuring the patient's safety and our own moral stability. Although we may not control the dying process itself or its timing, we can ensure a prompt and effective response to the needs of the patient and the patient's family by attending closely to what is happening.

If attending to the dying process is the object of the game of terminal care, what are the rules? If the dying process has no set pattern, how can we know where we stand? Three components make up this idea, and the smaller segments help us evaluate the terminal care we deliver (see table 2).

Rule 1: Invite Participation

Terminal care is not a game that should be played alone. That we expect death already makes us different from those around us in the hospital environment, and fighting this isolation is important. We can call on the chaplain, the social worker, and our colleagues for support. As clinicians, we have a certain amount of both power and powerlessness in this situation, and both should be shared.

Sharing the Power. Any previous experience with dying patients and nurses' relative emotional distance from the patient give us an advantage, compared with the patient's family members. We must

**Table 2. The Object of the Game and the Rules
for Terminal Care in the Intensive Care Unit**

Object of the game	Dying is a process, and attending to the dying process is an ethical end in itself.	
Rule 1	Invite participation.	Share the power and the powerlessness.
Rule 2	Allow time to pass.	Let the patient call the game.
Rule 3	Allow for unpredictability.	Complete control is neither possible nor desirable.

communicate what we know about the effects of the withdrawal of life support, helping the dying patient's family members understand what parts of the process they can expect to see and which parts are difficult to predict. We can invite the family members to share their preferences in the management of the dying process and offer them choices about whether they wish to be present or absent and to accommodate any religious or cultural observances that they prefer.

Sharing the Powerlessness. Certainly, we regret our inability to alter the ultimate outcome for the dying patient, and we cannot take away the family's grief. The dying process itself is not subject to our domination. If we can talk about these facts with one another, they may be easier to bear.

Rule 2: Allow Time to Pass

The patient gets to "call" the game, including how long it lasts. The interval between the time that life support is withdrawn and the time the patient dies may allow important work to be done. The patient's family members have the opportunity to say their good-byes and to talk about how things used to be and what the patient's life has meant to them. Family members can observe the physiological changes that signal the coming of death. In these ways, family members mark the significance of the patient's life and confirm for themselves not only how sick the patient has been but also that the patient's death was not hastened. Family members can prepare themselves for life without the patient's physical presence.

Rule 3: Allow for Unpredictability

We recognize that the most important "player" in the game has never died before. In making room for the unexpected, we are respecting the dignity of the patient and allowing the patient's dying to have its own style. Following this rule can be a fine line to walk. Although we want to give the patient enough medication to prevent unnecessary discomfort, our titration of medications should be governed by our assessment of the patient's condition at frequent intervals, rather than by a desire to preempt anything unpleasant.[22] A felt need to control is part and parcel of the territory of death itself,[23] along with feelings of helplessness, guilt, and vulnerability. Our experience in working in the ICU likewise predisposes us to discomfort when we lack control. We need reassurance that death (like birth) happens in its own time and in its own fashion. Too much control of the dying process gets us into ethical trouble, for we have the means at the bedside (unlike most hospice clinicians) consciously or unconsciously to hasten a patient's death.[24] Accordingly, if we are ill at ease because unpredictable things seem to be happening, it may be an indication that something ethically appropriate is taking place.

Summary

These three rules provide a means to evaluate our terminal care. If we are (1) inviting participation and communicating about the process of dying, (2) allowing time to pass, and (3) making room for the unexpected, then our attention to the dying process contains the appropriate qualities.

Attending to the dying process focuses especially on the interval between the withdrawal of life support and the patient's death. But just as the process of dying truly began before we implemented the decision to withdraw life support, our attention to it does not begin only when we extubate or stop the administration of vasopressors. Our intention to manage the dying process well requires attention to the preliminaries. The transition from football to baseball is a critical juncture, and our success at the new game depends on the groundwork we lay before the first pitch crosses the plate (see figure 1).

BETWEEN THE DECISION AND THE IMPLEMENTATION: LAYING OUT THE PLAYING FIELD

Although nursing excellence[25] is important throughout the dying process, the interval that comes between the decision to withdraw life support and its actual implementation can be particularly amenable to the influence of nurses, because they lay out the playing field for the new game of baseball. By influencing the quality of the transition from curative treatment to end-of-life care, nurses set the tone for what follows.

The game will run more smoothly if the field for the new game contains the following three elements:

- *Ethical consensus.* Everyone with a moral stake in the case should be in agreement that the withdrawal of life support and expected death is the appropriate outcome for the patient (consider case report 3).
- *Clinical consensus.* The team members and the family (and the patient, if appropriate) must be clear on their game plan for the patient. Nurses must encourage physicians to broaden the discussion to include the preferences of the patient and the patient's family in these matters, respecting each patient's style of death as much as the patient's style of life.[26] Patients may be receiving a number of therapies that

are considered life sustaining, including dialysis, antibiotics, and mechanical ventilation. If terminal care is to be centered on the patient and the patient's family, then biases of the physician regarding the order of withdrawal and the speed of the death[27] should not necessarily take precedence. If death by neurological criteria is a factor in the withdrawal of ventilatory support, how and when will the criteria be met? Do delays exist that can be planned for (e.g., arrival of family members, preparation of the morphine infusion)? If the unit has no protocol, in what order will the elements of life support be withdrawn?[28] These and other issues must be settled by the healthcare team with input from the patient's family before the process begins.

* *A comfortable patient and the means to maintain comfort.* Not only are appropriate orders from a physician necessary, but a nurse must also be available to titrate medication according to the patient's response.[29] In practical terms, this requirement means that the ICU may have to arrange coverage for the nurse's other patients.

These three elements must be ensured before withdrawal of life support begins. The responsibility for overseeing these arrangements lies with the nurse.

The decision to withdraw life support from a patient and the onset of a terminal-care perspective bring profound changes in focus. The normal hierarchy of orders given and carried out gives way to shared decision making among the clinicians, the patient's family, and the patient (if able). Instead of seeing the patient as an assembly of broken body systems, like Humpty Dumpty, we try to put the patient back together in our minds and treat him or her as a whole person, whose physical participation in a family and a community is about to be lost forever. We must open our tight universe of discrete medical interventions to holistic patient care and unlimited visitation.[30]

Nurses who orchestrate this consummate transition may feel pressed for time. Football is all around them, and the tolerance for a different game played in the same space may be low. How do they buy the time they need to set the proper tone? Remembering the following phrase, which is a combination of "Stop, Look, and Listen," and "Look, Listen, and Feel," may be helpful (see table 3): "Stop, Look, Listen, and Feel."

The environment of the ICU, its pace, and its penchant for control all mitigate against the possibility that Nature will take its course after the decision is made to withdraw life support from a patient. A reliance on "comfort care only" can skew our perspective when we consider our ethical obligations to dying patients. Dying patients deserve a broad vision of terminal care that reflects the hospice philosophy of a good death, even though the circum-

---

CASE REPORT 3

The intensive care unit is full. Mrs. D is an eighty-year-old woman admitted the day before with subarachnoid hemorrhage. She experiences sudden hypotension at 10 P.M. and requires dopamine and fluids for stabilization. The neurosurgery resident goes to the waiting room to inform Mrs. D's family of the change in her condition. On his return to the unit, the resident unexpectedly orders Mrs. D to be extubated and given "comfort care only." The respiratory therapist loosens the tape of the endotracheal tube in preparation for extubation. Meanwhile the nurse goes to the waiting room to discuss the withdrawal procedure with the family and ask about their preferences. The patient's family members express complete surprise and dismay at the prospect of extubation, saying that they understood only that no chest compressions would be used. The nurse returns and is relieved to find that Mrs. D has not been extubated. Inquiry reveals that the resident spoke with the son, the decision maker in the case, who then left the area to

---

Table 3. Stop, Look, Listen, and Feel

When the decision is made to stop curative treatment:

Stop   Take a "time-out" to think things through.

Look   Look at the big picture. This is the only time that this patient will ever die. What should happen? Who should be involved?

Listen   Listen to the patient's family and to the patient. What do they want to happen?

Feel   Feel how different this practice is from routine care in the intensive care unit.

stances of hospices and those of ICUs differ substantially. By orchestrating the transition from a curative to a palliative focus, nurses can lay the groundwork that enables the clinicians to attend to the dying process.

make telephone calls. The nurse spoke with two female members of the family who may or may not have been present for the conversation with the resident. Several hours later, the patient's family agrees to withdraw life support. Mrs. D dies early the next morning with seven family members gathered around her bed.

Case discussion: Although technically the resident had obtained consent from the appropriate person for withdrawal of life support, the lack of understanding and agreement discovered by the nurse was ethically relevant. Total agreement of far-flung family members to a treatment plan is not required by law, but the family members waiting together at the hospital late at night show their concern for the patient and thereby their moral standing in the case. Without an assent to withdrawal of life support from the family members she spoke to, the nurse could not allow the process to go forward. Had the nurse carried out the resident's order without investigation, a disastrous surprise might have awaited the family with the next visit.

NURSING AND TERMINAL CARE

Nurses find a way to play baseball on their football fields and deliver expert nursing care for their dying patients,[31] despite the lack of universal standards, formal death education, or mechanisms for accountability. Critical care nurses have always been able to bring the caring touch that humanizes the technology used, and many families report that the nursing care they and their loved one received around the death made a terrible event easier to bear.[32] This excellence, however, is practitioner-dependent and inconsistent. Much of the blame for this unevenness falls on the environment of acute care itself, which is organized to stabilize every patient's condition, without exception, and to keep moving to the next task. Hospitals are trying to overcome a reputation as the place where people go to die, and so terminal care has become a secret game in which no one keeps score except the family.

Change is at hand, however. The lack of universal protocols and standards for the hands-on management of end-of-life care is a void that current developments in palliative care and reimbursement policies are sure to fill.[33] Any nurse who cares for dying patients must use his/her influence to ensure that those patients receive appropriate, ethically responsible care. "Among all healthcare professionals, nurses have traditionally been the ones who try to bridge the gap between aggressive treatment interventions and holistic, compassionate care for patients at the end of life."[34] Nurses' advocacy should include teaching fellow clinicians about appropriate pain control, inviting participation from the patient's family members, and allowing the dying process to unfold, just as colleagues in hospice nursing have been doing in home care. The voices of nurses must help define not only the elements of excellence in terminal care but also the object of the game.

NOTES

1. "Measuring quality of care at the end of life: A statement of principles," Last Acts [online], www.lastacts.org/measurin.htm [29 July 1997].

2. D. F. Chambliss, *Beyond Caring: Hospitals, Nurses, and the Social Organization of Ethics* (Chicago: University of Chicago Press, 1996), pp. 8, 75–79, 165.

3. Ibid.

4. D. A. Asch, "The role of critical care nurses in euthanasia and assisted suicide," *N Engl J Med* 334 (1996): 1347–79; P. A. Ubel and D. A. Asch, "Semantic and moral debates about hastening death: A survey of bioethicists," *J Clin Ethics* 8 (1997): 242–49.

5. W. C. Wilson et al., "Ordering and administration of sedatives and analgesics during the withholding and withdrawal of life support from critically ill patients," *JAMA* 267 (1992): 949–53.

6. SUPPORT Principal Investigators, "A controlled trial to improve care for seriously ill hospitalized patients," *JAMA* 274 (1995): 1594–98; J. Lynn et al., "Perceptions by family members of the dying experience of older and seriously ill patients, *Ann Intern Med,* 126 (1997): 97–106; SUPPORT Investigators, "Study to understand prognoses and preferences for outcomes and risks of treatment," Inter-University Consortium for Political and Social Research, Study no. 2957; J. Addington-Hall, M. Lay, D. Altmann, and M. McCarthy, "Symptom control, communication with health professionals and hospital care of stroke patients in the last year of life as reported by surviving family, friends, and officials," *Stroke* 26 (1995): 2242–48.

7. C. A. Hite and M. F. Marshall, "Death and dying," in *Introduction to Clinical Ethics,* 2d ed., ed. J. C. Fletcher et al. (Frederick, Md.: University Publishing Group, 1997), pp. 127–54.

8. K. Turner et al., "Dignity in dying: A preliminary study of patients in the last three days of life," *J Palliat Care* 12 (summer 1996): 7–13.

9. H. Brody et al., "Withdrawing intensive life-sustaining treatment: Recommendations for compassionate clinical management," *N Engl J Med* 336 (1997): 652–57; C. K. Cassel and B. C. Vladeck, "ICD-9 code for palliative or terminal care," *N Engl J Med* 335 (1996): 1232–33; J. Lynn,

"Caring at the end of our lives," *N Engl J Med* 335 (1996): 201–202; Council on Scientific Affairs, AMA, "Good care of the dying patient," *JAMA* 275 (1996): 474–78; C. J. Marsden et al., "End-of-life care: Ethical dimensions, a continuing education monograph for nurses," Helix-On-Line Nursing CE Courses [online], www.helix.com/member/coned/nurse [29 August 1997].

10. W. Woolley, "AMA issues bill of rights for dying," *Detroit News* [online], www.detnew.com/1997/nation/9706/23/06230106.htm [23 June 1997].

11. "Measuring quality of care at the end of life: A statement of principles."

12. ACCP/SCCM Consensus Panel, "Ethical and moral guidelines for the initiation, continuation, and withdrawal of intensive care," *Chest* 97 (1990): 949–58; American Thoracic Society, "Withholding and withdrawing life-sustaining treatment," *Am Rev Respir Dis* 144 (1991): 726–31; Task Force on the Ethics of the Society for Critical Care Medicine, "Consensus report on the ethics of forgoing life-sustaining treatments in the critically ill," *Crit Care Med* 18 (1990): 1435–39.

13. C. Scanlon, "Defining standards for end-of-life care," *Am J Nurs* 97 (1997): 58–60.

14. M. L. Campbell, "Terminal weaning: It's not simply 'pulling the plug,'" *Nursing* 24 (1994): 34–39; M. E. Shekleton et al., "Terminal weaning from mechanical ventilation: A review," *AACN Clin Issues* 5 (1994): 523–33; B. J. Daly, D. Thomas, and M. A. Dyer, "Procedures used in withdrawal of mechanical ventilation," *Am J Crit Care* 5 (1994): 38–39.

15. L. Kirkland, "Neuromuscular paralysis and withdrawal of mechanical ventilation," *J Clin Ethics* 5 (1994): 38–39; C. H. Rushton and P. B. Terry, "Neuromuscular blockade and ventilator withdrawal: Ethical controversies," *Am J Crit Care* 4 (1995): 112–15.

16. J. A. Billings and S. D. Block, "Slow euthanasia," *J Palliat Care* 12 (1996): 21–30; K. Faber-Langendoen and D. M. Bartels, "Process of forgoing life-sustaining treatment in a university hospital: An empirical study," *Crit Care Med* 20 (1992): 570–77.

17. Joint Commission on Accreditation of Healthcare Organizations, "Standards, intents, and examples for patient rights" in *Comprehensive Accreditation Manual for Hospitals* (Oakbrook Terrace, Ill.: JCAHO, 1996 and quarterly updates), pp. RI6–RI13.

18. E. M. McGee, "Can suicide prevention in hospice be ethical?" *J Palliat Care* 13 (1997): 27–33.

19. Chambliss, *Beyond Caring*, pp. 8, 75–79, 165.

20. F. G. Miller and J. J. Fins, "A proposal to restructure hospital care for dying patients," *N Engl J Med* 334 (1996): 1740–42.

21. P. Ramsey, *The Patient as a Person* (New Haven, Conn.: Yale University Press, 1970).

22. G. G. Weatherill, "Pharmacologic symptom control during the withdrawal of life support: Lessons in palliative care," *AACN Clin Issues* 6 (1995): 344–51.

23. R. Kastenbaum, "In control," in *Psychosocial Care of the Dying Patient*, ed. C. A. Garfield (New York: McGraw-Hill, 1978), pp. 227–40.

24. Wilson et al., "Sedatives and analgesics," pp. 949–53.

25. S. D. McClement and L. F. Degner, "Expert nursing behaviors in care of the dying adult in the intensive care unit," *Heart Lung* 24 (1995): 408–19.

26. K. A. Koch, H. D. Rodeffer, and R. L. Wears, "Changing patterns of terminal care management in an intensive care unit," *Crit Care Med* 22 (1994): 233–43.

27. N. A. Christakis and D. A. Asch, "Biases in how physicians choose to withdraw life support," *Lancet* 243 (1993): 642–46.

28. D. A. Asch and N. A. Christakis, "Why do physicians prefer to withdraw some forms of life support over others? Intrinsic attributes of life-sustaining treatments are associated with physicians' preferences," *Med Care* 34 (1996): 103–11.

29. Brody et al., "Withdrawing intensive life-sustaining treatment," pp. 652–57.

30. Ibid.

31. S. D. McClement and L. F. Degner, "Expert nursing behaviors in care of the dying adult in the intensive care unit," *Heart Lung* 24 (1995): 408–19.

32. M. M. Furukawa, "Meeting the needs of the dying patient's family," *Crit Care Nurse* 16 (February 1996): 51–57.

33. Lynn et al., "Perceptions by family members"; SUPPORT Investigators, "Study to understand prognoses and preferences for outcomes and risks of treatment."

34. Scanlon, "Defining standards," pp. 58–60.

4

BEYOND
"DEATH with DIGNITY"
A Hospice Vignette

Douglas MacDonald

*S*ometime in August 1999 . . .

I'm sitting in another living room in another home of another family whose loved one is actively dying.

The nurse and I drove here, knowing that the gentleman was probably "imminent." We were here just yesterday afternoon, explaining the hospice program to his wife and two daughters. We discussed all the familiar "stumbling blocks," those issues that frequently delay people from accepting hospice services until it is too late.

The gentleman, whom I'll call Mr. Smith, has a feeding tube, and now his feedings are causing him to throw up continually, because his body can no longer accept the fluid and nutrition. We recommended discontinuing them. Mr. Smith has received periodic injections of Lupron, which sometimes slows the progression of prostate cancer. It is clear to us that this expensive therapy will no longer buy this eighty-one-year-old man any more time. We

Reprinted from *American Journal of Hospice & Palliative Care* 17, no. 2 (March/April 2000): 78–79.

recommended that the injections be stopped. In the past, when Mr. Smith had episodes of seizure activity, the family called 911 and the emergency medical technicians (EMTs) would transport him to the hospital. By the time the EMTs got there, the seizures were usually over. We recommended that the family call hospice instead of the ambulance when seizures began.

All of this was a bit more than Mr. Smith's family could process a day ago. They needed time to discuss our recommendations and our philosophy of "comfort care only" among themselves. They were 85 percent ready for hospice—clearly, they loved this man and did not want his suffering to continue—but the remaining 15 percent kept us away until now. After a "bad night," they called us back, and we are here to set up some services that will ease this man through the last hours of his life.

Technically, we could have been here six months ago. Patients are allowed to have hospice care when they are terminally ill, have a probable life expectancy of six months, and are not receiving curative medical treatment. However, people rarely consider hospice care six months before they die. If they are not in active treatment—receiving chemotherapy, radiation, or surgery—they are almost always in active denial, and the last thing they want to hear about is how well hospice will take care of them when they are bed-bound, incontinent, and in severe pain.

With all that I know after fifteen years as a hospice social worker, I doubt that I'll want to hear about it either.

Dying stinks! It is messy, painful, exhausting, and endlessly humiliating. "Death with dignity" is the hospice's motto, but it is hard to square what typically happens when we die with any familiar notion of dignity. What is "dignified" about losing all control of your bodily functions, wearing diapers like an enormous baby, becoming delirious and disoriented, smelling of urine, feces, and necrosis, and looking both unrecognizably bloated with edema and, at the same time, so wasted and shrunken that your dentures will no longer fit into your mouth?

In my view, "death with dignity" is about putting on your best suit while you can still wear it, writing a graceful and conciliatory note while you can still hold a pen, and then putting a gun to your head while you can still pull the trigger.

The National Hospice Organization (NHO) is adamantly opposed to suicide, assisted or otherwise, and there are many excellent reasons *not* to die in the fashion I've just described. However, "dignity" is not one of them.

When we stepped into the bedroom that morning, Mr. Smith looked like many dying cancer patients that I've seen: very pale, mouth opened, breathing rapidly, phlegm rattling nosily in his throat. My mother looked like this when she was dying in the hospital, only worse. She fell flat on her face when she suffered her fatal stroke and got two enormous, swollen, black eyes. My fastidious, witty, feisty, stylish mom took her final breath looking like a panda bear.

We have ordered Levson drops for the throat secretions, Roxanol for pain and easier breathing, and Ativan for restlessness and anxiety. Mr. Smith's wife and daughters know we are a phone call away, day or night. They know a nurse will visit the next day, or sooner if necessary. They know about our bereavement program. Now they are gathered around the bed, their eyes bright with tears, their voices soft and comforting, their smiles warm. They have been taking excellent care of him. If Mr. Smith can no longer afford dignity, at least he has his family to console him for its loss. That is about the most any of us can hope for, in such circumstances—and it is probably enough.

5

WHAT'S IN A NAME?

Bruce H. Chamberlain

As practitioners of end-of-life care, our message to physicians and the public is that patients, and families of patients, with terminal illness have special needs that should be addressed. We offer hospice as a means to meet these unique needs with skilled management of end-of-life symptoms as well as spiritual and emotional comfort and support. Yet, despite the apparent clarity of the message, the term *hospice* has become synonymous in the minds of many people, both lay and medical, with giving up, failure, and imminent death. Clearly, the message is not being heard.

In a situation where the message being delivered is so different from the message being received, some explanation for the discontinuity in meaning must be sought. With respect to hospice, poor benefit utilization and declining lengths of stay on service in the face of a truly remarkable Medicare entitlement bespeaks such a miscommunication.

The search for the cause of this problem seems to have settled

Reprinted from *American Journal of Hospice & Palliative Care* 18, no. 6 (November/December 2001): 81–82.

on the word *hospice* itself. Most of us have had the experience of presenting end-of-life care options to a patient, only to see the term *hospice* evoke such an emotional response that no further meaningful information can be communicated. Based on this observation, it has been suggested that the word is at the root of the communication problem; and so minimizing use of the word should resolve the miscommunication. This logic prompted the recent recommendation at the 2nd Joint Clinical Conference and Exposition on Hospice and Palliative Care[1] that providers of hospice care underplay the use of the word *hospice* in their activities. Perhaps the use of a new term such as "end-of-life care," or even usurping another name, such as "palliative care," will overcome the communication barrier that keeps hospice from joining the mainstream of accepted and acceptable care options. Some agencies have made a conscious decision to omit the term *hospice* from their name for this very reason. Yet, regardless of what we may choose to call ourselves, hospice is what we are and hospice care is what we provide; though a housewife may be called a "domestic engineer," she still dusts and cares for the children. I expect that the results of such a name change would be that of most euphemisms applied with the sole purpose of improving image; the new term would simply become an ironic parody of the original. Any new term we choose will certainly come to acquire the same meaning as the old one if the thing itself remains unchanged.

Another consideration might be that the fault for our public relations problem is not in the name at all; perhaps the problem lies deeper in the nature of the thing that the name represents, the hospice industry itself. Changing names is relatively easy compared with the painful introspection that really needs to occur for us to uncover the cause of the problem.

Given that the Medicare Hospice Benefit offers such a broad array of benefits and services for the terminally ill and their families, why has it come to have such a poor reputation? Why would a neurosurgeon in a local hospital tell the family of his patient who has just suffered a catastrophic hemorrhagic stroke: "The internist may recommend hospice care for your mother, but you don't want to involve them"? Do we honestly believe that he is intentionally depriving the family of an entitlement that will make this process easier, an entitlement for which the patient has already paid? Are there really that many physicians out there who would consciously choose not to provide these services for their patients, just because they view their patients' pending death as a personal failure, or because they are uncomfortable with the use of morphine? Is poor survival prognosticating on the part of attending physicians the only significant reason for late hospice referrals? Can we safely lay the bulk of the blame on preconceived and inaccurate perceptions of the word *hospice*, or should we consider expanding our differential diagnosis?

Among the services included in the Medicare Hospice Benefit are the following: "Medical supplies and appliances including drugs and biological, provided as needed for the palliation and management of the terminal illness and related conditions." The *Hospice and Palliative Medicine: Core Curriculum and Review Syllabus* says:

> Radiation, chemotherapy, surgery, and other aggressive palliative measures have appropriate uses in hospice and palliative medicine, as long as the goal of therapy is symptom relief, and the benefits of treatment outweigh the burdens . . . all treatment options are explored and evaluated within the context of the patient's wishes and the goals of care.[2]

I have seen statistics that show a large majority of agencies give lip service to providing these services, but the reality is that far too many do not.

A market analysis performed in more than thirty sites around the country, wherein hospice providers were called and presented with a fictional, scripted case scenario under the guise of seeking assistance for a sick parent, provided some disturbing information.[3] Some 47 percent of agencies required a patient to stop total parenteral nutrition (TPN) before admission and 41 percent required a patient to stop palliative chemotherapy or radiation therapy in order to be admitted. In this latter category, two large, multisite agencies refused admission 67 percent and 80 percent of the time unless the treatments were discontinued. Far too often, patients who meet eligibility criteria for hospice admission are refused access to their benefits because they have chosen to receive aggressive, palliative therapy. Some agencies are even more egregious in refusing antibiotics or intravenous (IV) fluid to patients who desire them. When patients or families call an agency and are told: "Call back when you are done with the treatment," "We can't admit you until you are ready to have a DNR," or "We don't accept patients who are on IVs," should we really be surprised that they come away with the perception that hospice means no treatment?

The Medicare Hospice Benefit is one of the most unique among government entitlements in that it allows providers to determine the types of treatments they will give, within the conditions of participation, based on the "philosophy" of the agency. This means agencies that have made a philosophic determination, for whatever reason, not to provide these types of treatments are not violating the conditions of participation in refusing to admit patients who desire those treatments. However, they are wrong if they choose to justify their choices, in presenting them to patients or physicians, as based on "Medicare regulations," thereby discouraging further investigation. They are also wrong when they fail to refer such patients to other hospice agencies, if available, that provide the desired services.

Finally, there are many agencies that routinely refuse admission to patients who will not have a Do Not Resuscitate (DNR) order. This is not only wrong, but also in violation of the law, which specifically prohibits conditioning admission on whether or not a patient has executed an advance directive.[4] The result of such misinformation is further perpetuating the image of "hospice—a last resort for the dying."

The potential financial implications of providing all the desired palliative interventions are daunting. The Medicare Hospice Benefit was not written with some of today's commonly used and very expensive medications and treatments in mind. There are two possible ways to make a meaningful impact on the cost issue. First, we need to work together as an industry to document the costs of providing reasonable palliative care as a means to justify an increase in the reimbursement rate. Second, by providing care and dispelling the myth of hospice as giving up, we will be able to acquire patients earlier in the course of the illness when the cost of care is often not so great and thereby disperse the costs over a longer length of stay. Smaller agencies may not have the option to provide high-intensity palliative care at current reimbursement rates. In that circumstance, disclosing the limitation as an agency's philosophy of care, rather than contributing to the already prevalent misinformation of a limit imposed by Medicare, will contribute to better community understanding of the hospice benefit.

For the patient, the patient's family, and the referring physician, it is not enough that we "care" or that we have chaplains, social workers, volunteers, physicians, nurses, and aides committed to help them through the dying process. It is not enough that we have lofty ideals and philosophy about the care of the dying patient. The problem with our message is that while, as an industry, we say one thing, in practice we often do something very different. No matter how loud we shout that hospice is not just giving up, as long as we require our patients to give up, we will not be heard. It will only be when we, as an industry, commit to and actually allow the type of palliative interventions that the terminally ill may need, or, within reason, want, that we will ever begin to dispel the widely held negative perceptions of hospice. It does not really matter what we choose to be called; a food service specialist still waits on tables.

NOTES

1. National Hospice and Palliative Care Organization, American Academy of Hospice and Palliative Medicine, Hospice & Palliative Nursing Association: 2nd Joint Clinical Conference and Exposition on Hospice and Palliative Care, Orlando, Florida, 23–26 March 2001.

2. American Academy of Hospice and Palliative Medicine, *Hospice and Palliative Medicine: Core Curriculum and Review Syllabus* (Dubuque, Iowa: Kendall/Hunt, 1999), p. 8.

3. "Strategic link survey of hospice providers," unpublished, 1999.

4. Department of Health and Human Services, *Advance Directives and Do Not Resuscitate (DNR) in Medicare Hospice Clarification* (Rockville, Md.: United States Government Printing Office, 2000).

Part Two

PALLIATIVE CARE AT THE END OF LIFE

6

A CAREGIVER'S QUANDARY
How Am I to Evaluate and Respond to the Other's Suffering?

Clyde Nabe

One of the incentives for the development of the modern hospice movement was the belief that the care provided sick persons not only often failed to deal effectively with their suffering[1] but that it sometimes even failed to recognize that suffering. Suffering persons might be told that they could not be having as much discomfort as they claimed. In other words, the persons' suffering was simply denied. Or they might be told that their suffering could not be alleviated because it would require the use of therapies (usually medications) that would produce undesirable outcomes (usually an addiction).

Hospice and palliative care theory have contributed to and improved the understanding, evaluation, and treatment of many sorts of pain. For instance, it has been established that suffering people do not need either to be in (even great) physical pain or to be unconscious. Instead, analgesia is the goal and hospice theory claims that this status is almost always realizable.[2] This outcome is

Reprinted from *OMEGA—Journal of Death and Dying* 39, no. 2 (1999): 71–81.

generally to be admired. However, there is a subtle danger lurking here. In a culture in which a technological imperative is often assumed,[3] that imperative provides at least implicit support to the belief that if something can be done, then it should be done. Thus, given the improved capabilities of alleviating pain, instead of erring on the side of inuring themselves to someone's suffering, caregivers may become oversensitive to that suffering. When this oversensitivity is combined with a view that suffering is evil, caregivers may believe that one should always intervene to end it.[4] However, this belief risks encouraging caregivers to ameliorate someone's suffering even if that closes off possibilities that are important to the suffering person.[5]

Robert Fulton addressed this issue when he wrote:

> The hospice directive . . . instructs us to relieve pain and to provide succor. This directive has been interpreted to embrace the relief of physical as well as spiritual pain. Presently, we struggle to find the proper stance to take with respect to what is appropriate for the sake of the soul and what is deserving of the flesh. We can see this struggle expressed in a recent directive from the Catholic Church which . . . reasserted the right, if not the spiritual desirability, of patients experiencing unrelieved death agonies in emulation of Christ.[6]

This article focuses on the issue of what one ought to do about suffering. There are at least three possible responses to this issue.

The first is that one should do nothing. Some have interpreted certain Christian teachings as implying that to alleviate suffering is to interfere with God's plan for the person.[7] The second reply takes the opposite position. It holds that one should always seek to alleviate and if possible even eliminate suffering. The third answer to the question holds that in some circumstances it is appropriate to intervene and in some circumstances it is not. This article argues that the most defensible answer to the question is the third one. That is, sometimes intervention to alleviate or eliminate suffering is appropriate and sometimes it is not. The article also offers some insight into how to distinguish between these two sorts of circumstances.

EVALUATING SUFFERING

This initial question is tied in important ways to a second one. What value is assigned to suffering? That is, what is the value of suffering in *itself*? There are four possible positions on this question: (1) suffering in itself is evil; (2) it is good; (3) in some situations it is evil, while in others it is good; (4) it is neither good nor evil. When something is called evil in this article, that means that one disapproves of it and that in turn means that one desires that it not be a part of one's experience. As Joel Kupperman put it, "[Suffering] is a state which, all things being equal, anyone would rather not have."[8] This will be enough for such a state to be called evil in this article and will be the only claim being made about that state when it is called evil. A state that is the opposite of this would here be called good. And a situation to which one is neither drawn nor from which one is repelled would be called a neutral situation. If something is neither good nor evil, then presumably neither are there any obligations to react to it in some specifiable manner. However, that suffering is neutral in this sense seems to be an unlikely position to take, so this view will not be addressed further in this article.

Perhaps most people would say that suffering in itself is evil. However, there are arguments made that suggest that at least under some circumstances it can be good. For instance, Adrian Caesar argued that in pre–World War I England, young men were taught that suffering was a part of being 'manly.' Since 'manliness' was viewed as a virtue in that culture, suffering as a part of that virtue was also thought to be good.[9]

The view that suffering can be good may also appear to be present in some Christian teachings. Consider the following statements. The first comes from a Roman Catholic document:

According to Christian teaching . . . suffering, especially suffering during the last moments of life, has a special place in God's saving plan; it is in fact a sharing in Christ's Passion and a union with the redeeming sacrifice which he offered. . . . Therefore one must not be surprised if some Christians prefer to moderate their use of painkillers, in order to accept voluntarily at least a part of their sufferings and thus associate themselves in a conscious way with the sufferings of Christ crucified.[10]

Writing from an Orthodox Christian perspective, Edward Hughes wrote:

Suffering is seen as a participation in Christ, and as such, is something to be desired rather than avoided. . . . The time "forced" upon (dying persons) near the end of their lives may be a great gift from God to those who sincerely need that time to discover and nurture their spirit. If we actively "liberate" them prematurely, before their spiritual work is done, we may deprive them of what God may have given them as the means to their salvation.[11]

In addition, John Edelman asked "why one resists calling suffering a good. I mean to point to the possibility that suffering can be a grace. If suffering can be a grace, then it can be seen as a gift from God."[12] He also wrote:

I am after a sense for the expression "Suffering is a grace" that is by no means identical to "Adversity builds character," at least if the latter is taken to mean that the value of the adversity or the suffering lies in the fact that it builds a kind of endurance that may be useful in the future.[13]

These claims seem to imply that suffering is not merely extrinsically good, but rather is good in itself.

However, the position taken in this article is (and others agree)[14] that suffering in itself is evil. Evidence that this is a reasonable position is found in the fact that we do not think it sensible

to congratulate or to encourage someone to undergo more suffering *merely for the sake of the suffering itself.*[15] If we encourage
someone to suffer, it is always to obtain some good external to the
suffering. That is, suffering is never intrinsically good. It is, at best,
a means to some desired end. In itself, it is undesirable. Even for
those who argue that suffering can lead to spiritual growth or to
some other desirable (for example, religious or psychological) consequences, positive value is located with that growth or those consequences, not in the suffering itself. Indeed, it is hard to imagine
why anyone would hold that suffering which led to no desirable
outcome was desirable in any way.

If this analysis is correct, then on its basis, a rough guideline of
when it may be appropriate and when it may be inappropriate to
oppose suffering is already available. If the evil of the suffering is
outweighed by the good associated with the end that is produced by
the means of the suffering, then it may be appropriate not to ameliorate the suffering. However, if the suffering is more evil than its
associated end is good, presumably that suffering can not be justified and that suggests that it should be ameliorated if possible.

Suffering has been claimed to be a means to many desirable
ends; among these are knowledge, wisdom, salvation, redemption,
greater emotional, moral and/or physical strength, artistic creativity, spiritual development, strength of character, strengthened
ties with other people, and the development of individual
autonomy.[16] Edelman drew attention to a particular sort of knowledge available only through the experience of suffering:

> There is an understanding that consists in the recognition of the
> limits of human power, and there is suffering that necessarily
> accompanies . . . this understanding, namely, the suffering—the
> pain—one feels in running up against those limits.[17]

These ends may all be desirable. But they do not justify suffering if they could be achieved by some means that did not involve
suffering. Those means would be preferred and should be chosen

instead. It is true that almost everyone on occasion uses means which have accompanying pain to achieve some end believed to be desirable. For example, we exercise—which in itself and as a consequence can produce pain—and we do this in order to achieve (at least in part) a healthier body (the desired end). And we demand that children engage in activities they do not want to perform (and thus may produce some suffering in them) in order to achieve certain goals: growth in maturity, education, moral probity. However, if we could get our children to learn mathematics or to develop writing skills without suffering, presumably only a sadistic parent or teacher would choose the means that included suffering.

Edelman's example is an important one because it illustrates a situation in which there are apparently no other means available—in principle—to achieve the desirable goal. However, two things need to be said about his example. The first is that it must be clear that the goal itself really is desirable. It is reasonable to ask why the knowledge described is desirable. If no case can be made for that claim, there would be no reason to pursue the goal. Second, even if knowledge of our limits is desirable, the desirability of such knowledge must outweigh the evil of the suffering that arises on the way to it and that is concomitant with it.

We might be able to construct an argument showing that this is the case. But such assessments are often notoriously difficult to make. In addressing a somewhat similar issue about the desirability of coming to recognize one's own capacity for evil, Eleonore Stump wrote:

> That natural evil and moral evil . . . serve to make men recognize their own evils . . . is a controversial claim; and it is dear that a compelling argument for or against it would be very difficult to construct. To produce such an argument we would need a representative sample, whatever that might be, of natural and moral evil. Then we would need to examine that sample case by case to determine the effect of the evil in each case on the human beings who suffered or perpetrated it. To determine the effect we would

have to know the psychological and moral state of these people both before and after the evil at issue ... and we would have to chart their state for the rest of their lives.[18]

This is an impressive, even daunting, set of tasks. And assessing spiritual growth or emotional maturity as well as many other of the recommended goals that usually have some suffering associated with their achievement seems unlikely ever to be accomplished in any thorough manner.

What does this mean for the claim that suffering may be acceptable if it leads to a desirable end? It means that the onus of the proof is on the person who makes the claim that this particular instance of suffering is outweighed by the desirability of that particular end.

In making such a judgment, it will often not be enough to argue that the evil tied to the class of some sort of suffering (say, the pain associated with terminal cancer) is outweighed by the good associated with some *class* of desirable ends (say, spiritual growth) supposedly achieved via that suffering. This is because suffering is always an individual matter.[19] The suffering that I experience associated with my lower back pain may be greater or lesser than the suffering another person experiences with her lower back pain. Rough estimates based on groups of people's experience often serve us well enough; for example, one can claim uncontroversially that almost all children are more benefitted by memorizing the multiplication tables than they are damaged by the suffering associated with that process. However, there are many other circumstances (for example, illness—perhaps especially terminal illness) where the sufferings are so complex and so interwoven with the unique personality, history, and circumstances of the individual involved that little success can be expected to be achieved by using generalizations about groups of people's experience.

WHO SHOULD MAKE THESE DECISIONS?

This leads to another question. Who is in the best position to judge that this suffering is outweighed by the end to be achieved? Most people believe that they know how to answer this question in at least one situation, that of children. As a general rule, adults are in a better position to determine that the suffering to be experienced by the child in order to reach a particular goal is outweighed by the desirability of that goal. Still, even this rule has exceptions; for instance, its application is dependent to some extent on the age and maturity of the individual child.

If we feel comfortable in our weighing of the associated suffering against the achievement of some desired goal in the case of children, what about adults? At first glance, it seems that only the individual involved is in a position to make such a judgment. After all, only I can assess the severity of my suffering; no one else can know it.[20] And as a general rule, this seems a wise position to take. It reduces the likelihood that one person may, based on ignorance, impose suffering on someone else. Persons are likely to evaluate suffering and desired ends in terms of their own values, and there is no reason to believe that one person's values on such intimate matters overlap in any precise way with another person's values. Thus, other persons are vulnerable to misassessing the suffering person's pain and values.

That the suffering person is best located to decide on the value of his or her suffering certainly seems to be the best position to take in the practice of medicine. This is especially true in the current situation, because instruction in the recognition of and proper assessment of suffering is so often missing in contemporary medical education.[21] If caregivers are not competent at recognizing and evaluating the significance of someone's suffering, they may make inappropriate decisions about the provision of care. However, as a court forcefully and, in my view, rightfully asserted in a related situation: "It is incongruous, if not monstrous, for medical practitioners to assert their right to preserve a life that someone else must live, or more accurately, endure."[22]

People sometimes decide that suffering, even if it is not a means to some desired end, is still acceptable for other reasons. Christine Longaker pointed this out when she wrote in the voice of dying people she had known:

> You may not know what it is like to live with constant pain and discomfort. What is hardest is when no one believes the amount of pain I am having. . . . I need to be believed and I need to have my pain relieved. But please don't knock me unconscious to do it. I would rather experience a little pain, and still be conscious . . . to do my spiritual practice—while I am in the last few weeks of my life (italics in original).[23]

People may choose to accept suffering not just to continue their spiritual practice, but also to visit loved ones, be at home rather than in an institution, or for many other reasons.

There is a difference between the situations just described and the ones discussed earlier. When suffering is understood to be a means to a desired end, it might be called "meaningful suffering." However, some suffering does not serve as a means to any end. It is just suffering per se and as such it might be called meaningless suffering. The arguments used earlier to show that some suffering may appropriately be unameliorated will not work for meaningless suffering. It is not an instance in which the desirability of the goal aimed at via the suffering outweighs the evil of that suffering.

Nevertheless, a similar weighing may be used here. While here the goal is not dependent on the suffering, again the desirability of the end being aimed at (for example, seeing one's loved ones in one's distant hometown) may outweigh the undesired suffering that will be occasioned by making the trip. Thus, even meaningless suffering may be accepted to achieve some desired goal. In such situations, again it would seem that the individual who will have to endure the suffering is the one best located to evaluate that suffering in reference to desired ends.

TROUBLESOME CASES

This leaves one last question: Is it ever the case that someone other than the suffering person is better located to make the decision about the value to be given to that person's suffering? This question has already been answered in the affirmative in the case of children. However, consider the following situations involving adults. (1) The first is one in which the suffering person's pain is a means to desirable ends for other persons. (2) The second is a situation in which a person other than the sufferer sees more or more clearly what the suffering can mean for the person in pain.

(1) Is it always outrageous to expect or even require that one person suffer in order to achieve the desired ends of someone else? The answer to this question is, of course, no. We do this in many situations: for example, with military service, quarantines, and vaccinations. Indeed most civil law is to one degree or another the imposition of some degree of suffering on one person for the benefit of others.

How far should this be taken? It is probably true that other people may achieve desirable ends by witnessing and dealing with someone's suffering. It is often claimed, for example, that family members and friends may learn something about themselves, about life and death, about courage and compassion by being present to a dying person's suffering. And this claim does not appear to be obviously unlikely to be true. Is this enough to justify not ameliorating that suffering?

(2) It is also probably true that there are situations in which some care providers may be better able to assess the relative value of an individual's suffering and the desirable outcomes that person may achieve either through or despite that suffering. Spiritual advisers may have traveled further along a spiritual path and thus know that to achieve greater spiritual growth one must pass through this suffering. Is this enough to justify not ameliorating this suffering?

One condition must be met before this second question can be answered in the affirmative. That condition is that the suffering must not be so great that it eliminates any reasonable expectation that any positive aim could be achieved.[24]

Even if this condition is met, however, there is no general rule to be applied in these situations. Rather, for both of the situations under discussion, to reach an appropriate decision requires that there be careful, attentive communication among the relevant persons. Decisions in these situations must be made on an individual, case by case, basis and must be based on careful reflection on the values and perceptions of the individuals involved.

A statement by the Roman Catholic Church should also be noted in reference to these last issues:

> It would be imprudent to impose a heroic way of acting as a general rule. On the contrary, human and Christian prudence suggest for the majority of sick people the use of medicines capable of alleviating or suppressing pain, even though these may cause as a secondary effect semiconsciousness and reduced lucidity. As for those who are not in a state to express themselves, one can reasonably presume that they wish to take these painkillers, and have them administered according to the doctor's advice.
>
> However, painkillers that cause unconsciousness need special consideration. For a person not only has to be able to satisfy his or her moral duties . . . he or she also has to prepare himself or herself with full consciousness for meeting Christ.[25]

Thus, even if one believes that heaven or hell, the vision of God, a more desirable reincarnation, or nirvana is at stake, caregivers must be wary of allowing someone to suffer in order to make possible some such achievement. However, the opposite danger must also be avoided. Dying persons may well decide to endure suffering—even an amount or form of suffering—with which caregivers find it difficult to live. However, even if a caregiver would not want to or believes that she or he could not tolerate the suffering another person is experiencing, it is no reason to intervene in that suffering if the sufferer chooses to accept that suffering for her or his own reasons.

No one is infallible in making these judgments. Therefore, strong measures of humility, compassion, and an openness to other persons are required when deciding what to do about someone's suffering if morally appropriate actions are to be taken. As Juliana Casey put it, those who care for suffering persons need an "exquisite sensitivity" to "and a profound respect" for those suffering persons.[26] When these virtues are realized, then caregivers will be more likely to help suffering persons instead of contributing to their suffering.

NOTES

1. In this article, the two terms *pain* and *suffering* are used interchangeably. While there may be good reasons to distinguish between them, no such distinction will be drawn here. [See E. J. Cassell, "The nature of suffering and the goals of medicine," *N Engl J Med* 306, no. 1 (1982): 639–45, and J. Shaffer, "Pain and suffering," in *Philosophical Dimensions of the Neuro-medical Sciences*, ed. S. F. Spicker and H. T. Engelhardt (Dordrecht, Germany: Reidel, 1976).] First of all, it will be assumed that the reasoning used in reference to suffering is applicable in a similar manner to pain. But as Erich Loewy notes, "Neither the literature of medicine nor the philosophical, sociological, and psychological literature deals with the concept of suffering in any stematic or thorough fashion." [See E. H. Loewy, *Suffering and the Beneficent Community: Beyond Libertarianism* (Albany: State University of New York Press, 1991).] And the few attempts to define suffering with or without reference to its relationship to pain have not been particularly convincing. These attempts have often ended up stipulating definitions for the concept, but the stipulated definitions fail to encompass all that people experience as and understand to be suffering. Suffering, as Loewy put it, is a "supple concept." [See Loewy, *Suffering and the Beneficent Community*, p. 4.] The truth is that suf-

fering is not a term that is easily defined; indeed Casey suggests that the attempt to define suffering is an "impossible task." [See J. Casey, "Suffering and dying with dignity," in *Suffering and Healing in Our Day*, ed. F. A. Eigo (Villanova, Penn.: Villanova University Press, 1990), pp. 137–66.]

2. R. Melzack, "The tragedy of needless pain," *Scientific American* 262, no. 2 (1990): 27–33; R. G. Twycross, *Symptom Management in Advanced Cancer* (New York: Radcliffe Medical Press, 1995).

3. D. Callahan, *The Troubled Dream of Life: In Search of a Peaceful Death* (New York: Touchstone, 1993); E. J. Cassell, *The Nature of Suffering and the Goals of Medicine* (New York: Oxford University Press, 1991).

4. Arthur Kleinman has drawn attention to this problem in the following way: "For many patients with serious, chronic conditions . . . suffering is a way of life. . . . The claims made for high technology interventions and the growth of our scientific knowledge base . . . hide that reality, as do the facile expectations that psychotherapy and psychopharmacology can relieve residual pain and suffering . . . the culture of biomedicine . . . (and) popular culture . . . have great difficulty coming to terms with the limits of treatment and the reality of suffering as a way of life. . . . Many Americans, together with increasing numbers of people in other affluent societies, seem to regard suffering as something that no one need feel, that one can and should avoid, that is without any redeeming virtue, and as something to which society should respond primarily with the high technology that defines our age." [See A. Kleinman, "Everything that really matters: Social suffering, subjectivity, and the remaking of human experience in a disordering world," *Harvard Theological Review* 90, no. 3 (1997): 315–35.]

5. P. Chidwick, *Dying, Yet We Live: Our Spiritual Care of the Dying* (Toronto: Anglican Book Center, 1988), pp. 41, 43, 58.

6. R. Fulton, "Commentary," in *Quest of the Spiritual Component of Care for the Terminally Ill*, ed. F. S. Wald (New Haven, Conn.: Yale University Press, 1986), p. 155.

7. L. Kumasaka, "My pain is God's will," *Amer J Nurs* 96, no. 6 (1996): 45–47; E. Stump, "The problem of evil," *Faith and Philosophy* 2, no. 4 (1985): 412.

8. J. Kupperman, "Suffering, joy, and social choice," *Public Affairs Quarterly* 8, no. 1 (1994): 51.

9. A. Caesar, *Taking It Like a Man: Suffering, Sexuality, and the War*

Poets: Sassoon, Owen, Graves (New York: Manchester University Press, 1993), p. 226.

10. SCDF, "Declaration on euthanasia," in *Vatican Council II: More Postconciliar Documents*, ed. A. Flannery (Grand Rapids, Mich.: William B. Eerdmans, 1982), p. 513–14. See also Matt. 72:34.

11. E. W. Hughes, "The act of death and the gift of suffering: A response to Breck, Amundsen, and Bresnahan, *Christian Bioethics* 1, no. 3 (1995): 342, 344.

12. J. T. Edelman, "Suffering and the will of God," *Faith and Philosophy* 10, no. 3 (1993): 382, 384.

13. Ibid., p. 384.

14. Chidwick, *Dying*, p. 43; Kupperman, "Suffering, joy, and social choice," p. 62; Loewy, *Suffering and the Beneficent Community*, p. 3; E. Stump, "The problem of evil," *Faith and Philosophy* 2, no. 4 (1985): 413.

15. Chidwick, *Dying*, p. 43.

16. J. Breck, "Euthanasia and the quality of life debate," *Christian Bioethics* 1, no. 3 (1995): 329; M. C. Rawlinson, "The sense of suffering," *J Med Phil* 11 (1986): 55–60; Kupperman, "Suffering, joy, and social choice," pp. 51, 52, 62; Stump, "The problem of evil," p. 411.

17. Edelman, "Suffering and the will of God," p. 383.

18. Stump, "The problem of evil," p. 409.

19. E. J. Cassell, "Recognizing suffering," *Hastings Center Report* (May–June 1991): 26; M. B. O'Brien, "Relief of suffering/Where the art and science of medicine meet," *Postgraduate Medicine* 99, no. 6 (1996): 189.

20. E. Scarry, *The Body in Pain: The Making and Unmaking of the World* (New York: Oxford University Press, 1985).

21. Cassell, "The nature of suffering," p. 639; Cassell, *The Nature of Suffering and the Goals of Medicine*, p. 32.

22. *Bouvia v. Superior Court*, 225 Cal 297, Cal.App.2Dist. (1986).

23. C. Longaker, *Facing Death and Finding Hope: A Guide to the Emotional and Spiritual Care of the Dying* (New York: Doubleday, 1997), p. 19.

24. Breck, "Euthanasia and the quality of life debate," pp. 329, 331; Rawlinson, "The sense of suffering," p. 57.

25. SCDF, "Declaration on euthanasia," pp. 513, 514.

26. Casey, "Suffering and dying with dignity," p. 158.

7

PALLIATIVE TREATMENTS OF LAST RESORT
Choosing the Least Harmful Alternative

Timothy E. Quill,
Barbara Coombs Lee, and Sally Nunn,
for the University of Pennsylvania
Center for Bioethics
Assisted Suicide Consensus Panel

Comprehensive palliative care, which includes pain and symptom management, support for patient and family, and the opportunity to achieve meaningful closure to life, is the standard of care for the dying.[1] Any intervention that is likely to hasten death should be considered only as a last resort, when life has become intolerable to the patient in the face of unrestrained efforts to relieve suffering.[2] In the United States, it is agreed that patients should receive sufficient treatment of their pain,[3] even at doses that risk hastening death, and that patients have the right to forgo life-sustaining treatment, even if their purpose is an earlier death.[4] Recently, terminal sedation and voluntary termination of eating and drinking have been proposed as legally acceptable alterna-

Reprinted from *Annals of Internal Medicine* 132 (2000): 488–93.

tives to physician-assisted suicide for persons whose suffering cannot be addressed by standard pain management and cessation of life support.[5] Outside of Oregon,[6] physician-assisted suicide remains illegal in the United States, although a covert practice exists in the rest of the country.[7] Because any of these acts could result in a hastened death, their moral and clinical evaluation should always consider the clinical context, the proportionate degree of suffering, the inadequacy of less drastic alternatives, and the nature of the decision-making process.[8]

When a patient expresses the wish to die, exploration of the adequacy of palliative care should begin, including assessment of pain management, depression, anxiety, family burnout, and spiritual and existential issues.[9] For patients who are genuinely ready to die, for whom suffering is intolerable despite comprehensive palliative efforts, an exploration of methods for easing death can begin. The methods will be determined by the patient's clinical situation; the values of the patient, family, and physician; and the status of current law. The table below outlines current methods that may hasten death. The first four options can be practiced openly, with good documentation and consultation, whereas the latter must be carried out covertly, except in Oregon.[10] Clinicians faced with these difficult decisions should be aware of all of these options, including their indications, risks, benefits, and likely outcomes, and how to discuss them with patients and families.

We present relatively straightforward clinical synopses of actual cases to illustrate how and when each of the interventions might be chosen. Each scenario is followed by a brief clinical commentary, with references for those who want to learn more about the legal, ethical, and policy implications and controversies. Knowledge of the availability of these options can be valuable to patients who have witnessed a bad death and fear a similar experience. Most persons will not request assistance in hastening death if they receive state-of-the-art palliative care, but some want to know that the potential for escape exists. Knowledge of the range

Table 1. Last-Resort Palliative Interventions

Intervention*	Certainty of Death	Patient Competence	Physician Involvement	Legal Status	Ethical Consensus
Standard pain management	Uncertain and unintended by patient or physician	Not required	Necessary	Legal	Yes
Forgoing life-sustaining therapy	Certain if dialysis is forgone; uncertain if ventilation, feeding tube, steroids, or insulin is forgone	Not required	Usually necessary	Legal	Yes
Voluntarily stopping eating and drinking	Certain, but requires time and discipline	Required	Desirable but not necessary	Legal	Growing consensus on its acceptability
Terminal sedation: heavy sedation to escape pain, shortness of breath, other severe symptoms	Certain if fluids are withheld (the standard practice)	Not required	Necessary	Legal	Growing consensus on its acceptability
Physician-assisted suicide†	Uncertain (patient may not take medication at all or not take as directed; medication may not work)	Required	Necessary for prescribing, unnecessary for administering	Illegal in all but one U.S. state, but unlikely to result in prosecution	No consensus on acceptibility but has considerable public support
Voluntary active euthanasia	Certain	Required	Necessary	Illegal and likely to be prosecuted	No consensus on acceptibility

*Options are listed in order of increasing legal and ethical uncertainty.

†We use the term "physician-assisted suicide" for clarity because of its widespread use in the medical literature, but we do not believe that the term "suicide" accurately reflects the meaning of this action, nor does it necessarily differentiate this practice from other last-resort practices. Technically, the last four practices might be considered suicide in the sense that death was sought by the patient as the only means of escaping intolerable suffering. However, the term "suicide" also connotes an act of self-destructiveness by a person with mental illness, whereas in each of these cases, death was viewed by the patients as a form of self-preservation. We must ensure that politicized public discussion about the legalization of physician-assisted suicide does not lead to distortion of the issues and ultimately to uninformed decision making.

of possibilities can also help clinicians better respond to the relatively rare patients whose pain and suffering become intolerable, without violating their own values and without abandoning their patients. Clinicians who care for severely ill patients must become aware of these options and decide which ones they are willing to provide as a last resort.[11] The challenge is to find the least harmful alternative given the patient's circumstances and the values of the patient, family, and clinicians involved.

CLINICAL EXAMPLES OF LAST-RESORT INTERVENTIONS

STANDARD PAIN MANAGEMENT

A sixty-eight-year-old man with metastatic small-cell lung cancer had excruciating bone pain and was near death. He initially responded to a combination of radiation and chemotherapy and had a three-year remission. When his disease recurred four months ago, he chose a palliative approach. His pain from extensive bony metastases was initially well controlled with high-dose, around-the-clock opioids supplemented by radiation and nerve blocks. He prepared for death through talks with his family and clergy, and he felt that he had no remaining "unfinished business." At that time, he weighed eighty pounds, he was bedbound, and his pain averaged eight points on a ten-point scale. He did not want to die but was willing to accept the risk for earlier death that might come from further increasing doses of opioids. After a palliative care consultation, his physician increased his total opioid doses by 25 percent per day until the pain was adequately controlled, or, if sedated, he appeared comfortable.

On the third day, the patient became very sleepy but arousable and appeared relatively free of pain. The physician shifted an equianalgesic amount of opioids from oral to transcutaneous administration because the patient was unable to reliably swallow. The patient became unresponsive but appeared comfortable, and he remained in that state until he died two days later.

COMMENTARY

Standard pain management has wide social acceptance by medical, legal, and religious groups and the public.[12] For most of his illness, this patient's pain was well controlled with high-dose opioids, and he was fully alert and functioning. When his pain increased toward the end of life, both patient and physician were willing to risk an earlier death as an unintended side effect, but it was neither a hidden nor an explicit purpose. The patient's suffering was proportionately severe enough to warrant taking the risk. Therefore, this action was consistent with the rule of double effect.[13] Had the patient's or the clinician's intent been to hasten death, it would be more difficult to use this rule to justify such treatment.[14] Although good pain management can usually be achieved without sedation and without shortening life, sometimes a patient's pain is so severe or the patient is so frail that the risk for accelerating death is real. When the patient in the above case study lapsed into a sedated state, the dose of opioid was neither increased nor decreased, and the side effect of sedation was accepted as proportionately necessary to control his pain.

WITHDRAWAL OF LIFE SUPPORTS

A fifty-six-year-old man developed a malignant brain tumor three years ago. He initially responded to a combination of surgery, radiation, chemotherapy, and corticosteroids. Although his cognitive abilities were diminished so that he could no longer work as an accountant, his altered brain unleashed new creativity in his hobby of painting. Later, when his tumor began to rapidly grow, he developed terrifying seizures during which he felt paranoid, confused, and attacked. During his seizure-free times, he talked in earnest about being ready to die. He was treated with anticonvulsants and antidepressants, with little relief. He tried unsuccessfully to end his life by jumping into Lake Ontario in winter; as a result, he was kept under twenty-four-hour supervision for being "suicidal."

The patient's physician subsequently realized that dexamethasone therapy was probably prolonging his life and that the patient could choose to discontinue it. After ethics and palliative care consultations, it was decided that it was both morally acceptable and clinically appropriate to provide this option to the patient, who immediately refused further dexamethasone. Within twelve hours, the patient went into a deep coma (probably from a combination of brain swelling and iatrogenic adrenal insufficiency). He had no pain or agitation and died peacefully twenty-four hours later.

COMMENTARY

The patient's right to refuse life-sustaining treatment, or to stop it once it has been started, has wide legal and ethical acceptance.[15] This right holds even if the patient wishes to die but could live indefinitely with treatment, provided that the patient is fully informed about the alternatives and has the mental capacity to understand the decision. Families can generally make these decisions on behalf of a patient who has lost mental capacity, provided there is a clear consensus that such actions reflect the patient's values, previously stated wishes, and best interests.[16] Because these decisions frequently result in the patient's death, clinicians should be forthright about evaluating such requests and carefully assess the patient's mental capacity, information about all palliative care alternatives, and the proportionate presence of suffering. This particular patient's wish to die was labeled as "suicidal" until it was realized that he was within his rights to stop life supports. This realization allowed a more open-minded conversation between patient, family, physicians, and the healthcare team than was previously possible.

Voluntary Termination of Eating and Drinking

An eighty-three-year-old woman was admitted to a nursing facility one year after experiencing a major cerebrovascular accident that left her with a dense hemiparesis but retained cognition. She stayed at home for the first year after her stroke with extensive support from her family and the visiting nurse service, but her skilled nursing needs eventually increased to the point that care at home was too difficult. Her other chronic medical problems included degenerative joint disease, osteoporosis, and coronary artery disease.

Six months after the admission, after extensive discussions with her family, her doctor, and clergy, the patient stopped taking all medicines other than pain relievers and adopted a purely palliative approach. Her care at the nursing facility was supplemented by a hospice team. Her goal was to achieve a quicker end to what had become, for her, an interminable dying process. She initially felt elated by the decision and began saying good-bye by telling her life story to her family in tape-recorded interviews. After three months of meaningful preparation, she had told all her stories, and her condition had again stabilized in what she viewed as a very poor quality of life.

The patient then began talking in earnest about wanting to die. Being a lifelong Unitarian, she had no personal moral objection to voluntarily hastening death, but she refused to compromise anyone in her family or her physician, given the current state of the law. She read a newspaper account of a woman who had chosen to stop eating and drinking,[17] and immediately began exploring this option with her family and physician. Her family initially worried that it would be a long, painful process, but her doctor found some reassuring data about patients with cancer who died in this way.[18] Several staff members were unable to accept her choice and were reassigned to other patients.

As the process unfolded, her family visited every day in rotating shifts. The patient was initially very talkative and had a special word for each of her children and grandchildren. On day six, she became sleepy and intermittently confused. The nursing staff kept her mouth moist and her skin well moisturized with lotion. Her favorite music played constantly in the background. The staff was prepared to provide sedation if she became agitated or clearly uncomfortable, but this proved unnecessary. She was in a coma for the final three days of the fifteen-day process.

COMMENTARY

Voluntarily stopping eating and drinking usually leads to death within one to three weeks.[19] Because the physician's role is indirect (ensuring an informed decision and awareness of palliative care alternatives, then addressing uncomfortable symptoms), this process does not require a change in the law. Because stopping eating and drinking is viewed as a variant of stopping life-sustaining treatment, it is in theory available to persons who do not have imminently terminal conditions. The process initially requires self-discipline and cooperation from family and healthcare providers. The substantial delay between initiation and death may be prohibitive for some patients with severe, immediate symptoms. Patients may also face additional challenges from symptoms that occur as the process unfolds. However, many patients who fear prolonged suffering and lack of choice find this possibility reassuring because it does not necessarily require "permission" from healthcare providers. In fact, especially if the patient is in a healthcare institution, the team must agree at a minimum not to interfere. Ideally, clinicians participate in the initial evaluation and then palliate symptoms throughout the course.

TERMINAL SEDATION

A thirty-five-year-old man had had AIDS for more than ten years. He had been near death several times over the past five years and had been in an AIDS hospice at the time when protease inhibitors became available. With the addition of protease inhibitors to his therapeutic regimen, the patient overcame recurrent infections and severe wasting and felt robust, gained weight, and returned to his work as a designer for two years. However, over the next nine months, his disease again began to progress in spite of numerous adjustments to his medication dose. He started losing weight, developed AIDS-related enteropathy, and began to lose his sight because of long-standing cytomegalovirus retinitis. This time, despite numerous changes in his antiretroviral regimen, he experienced no reprieve. The patient was again admitted to a residential hospice. He was very fearful of AIDS dementia and wanted to be reassured that he could be sedated if he became severely confused or agitated.

The patient's initial time in the hospice program was comfortable and meaningful because he had healing contact with family, friends, and clergy. As death approached, he developed high fevers, rigors, and increasing shortness of breath. These symptoms were treated with a morphine infusion and acetaminophen, but no medical workup was done and no antibiotic treatment was given. As the dose of morphine was increased to try to relieve his symptoms, the patient became delirious and agitated. When the dose was decreased the patient became more lucid but was very uncomfortable. He asked his doctor to help him escape from his agony. The doctor offered to sedate him to the point of unconsciousness and then withhold further treatment, including intravenous fluids. The patient was reassured that the sedative dose would be increased until he appeared to be resting comfortably and that it would not be cut back until he died. The healthcare team, the patient, and his family reached the consensus that this was the best of the available options. It would allow the patient to achieve the death that he wished for without violating the law or forcing him to suffer unnecessarily. He was given a midazolam infusion that was titrated upward until he achieved a sedated state and was then maintained at that level. He died within twenty-four hours.

COMMENTARY

Terminal sedation has been proposed as an alternative to physician-assisted suicide for terminally ill patients with severe symptoms. This method does not require changes in the law.[20] The patient is sedated to unconsciousness to relieve severe physical suffering and is then allowed to die of dehydration or some other intervening complication. Terminal sedation is ethically considered to be a combination of aggressive symptom management (sedatives to treat unbearable symptoms) and withdrawal of life-sustaining therapy (fluids, nutrition, and other treatments). When considered as an aggregate act, terminal sedation may be more morally complex and ambiguous than is generally acknowledged,[21] but many persons who adamantly oppose physician-assisted suicide find this practice acceptable.[22] The practice differs from euthanasia in that the dose of medication is maintained but not increased once sedation is achieved and no subsequent intervention to accelerate death, such as the introduction of a muscle-paralyzing agent, is given.

Terminal sedation allows healthcare providers to respond to a much wider range of suffering than would physician-assisted suicide even if it were legalized, because the latter would be restricted to competent terminally ill patients who are capable of self-administration. Terminal sedation has been used to respond to troubling syndromes such as terminal delirium, in which patients lose mental capacity at the end of life. The sedation itself is a mixed blessing—the patient is unaware of suffering but spends his or her last days in an iatrogenic coma. The facts that terminal sedation is not immediately lethal and requires a team to administer it are felt by some to be important safeguards. Guidelines for the practice of terminal sedation have been proposed,[23] but little is known about actual practice patterns.

PHYSICIAN-ASSISTED SUICIDE

A fifty-nine-year-old man received a diagnosis of oropharyngeal cancer two years ago. Because the tumor was too large to be resected, the patient was treated with chemotherapy and radiation. He was relatively asymptomatic for one year, during which he worked at his usual job. His tumor recurred inside his mouth and in his neck, making it hard to swallow his secretions. His initial goal was to live as long as his symptoms could be adequately managed and then to die as quickly and painlessly as possible. He was particularly afraid of suffocation, which he had seen in a coworker who died of emphysema. His pain was well controlled with around-the-clock administration of sustained-release morphine. After exploring his options, he was admitted to a home hospice program.

The patient's time on hospice was very meaningful, with regular visits from members of his church congregation, friends, hospice nurses, aides, and volunteers, in addition to his family. Unfortunately, his tumor eventually began to bleed profusely inside his mouth and outside his neck. He was terrified of suffocating and bleeding to death. He asked for enough barbiturates to "put me out of my misery." He considered stopping eating and drinking but felt the wait for death would be too long given his acutely deteriorating condition. He was offered terminal sedation so that he could escape his suffering, but he remained fearful of bleeding and suffocating but not being able to tell his caregivers about his subjective state. He was also worried about the impact that watching him bleed to death would have on his family. His family understood and accepted his decision and was willing to support him in the process if the physician would provide a prescription for barbiturates. After discussing the situation with his practice partners, the physician reluctantly but knowingly provided him with a lethal amount of barbiturates in a prescription ostensibly intended for insomnia. That evening, the patient took the entire amount with his family present, went into a deep sleep, and died quietly. Because the practice was illegal, the patient's final events were not documented.

COMMENTARY

This patient chose physician-assisted suicide because other last-resort options could not satisfactorily address his particular situation.[24] After a long period of excellent palliation, this patient's symptoms intensified greatly as death approached. Voluntarily stopping eating and drinking would not act quickly enough to respond to his particular clinical circumstances. Terminal sedation was also possible, but he feared suffocating while sedated and being unable to alert his caregivers of his distress. He was also concerned about the impact on his family were he to bleed to death while sedated. The physician, after having a private conversation about the clinical situation with his colleagues, reluctantly provided a prescription for barbiturates that could hasten death if taken all at once. Because of fear of legal action, the physician was not physically present to respond to complications but was available to the family by phone should problems arise. Maintaining the patient in a terminally sedated state was the physician's backup plan, but the patient died without complications.

DISCUSSION

Although the case studies presented here portray clear distinctions among the five last-resort interventions, in practice both the clinical indications and the practices may blur. Categorization may depend on specific circumstances and may be subject to interpretation. For example, the distinction between terminal sedation and voluntary active euthanasia is based in part on whether the dose of sedative is maintained or increased once sedation is achieved and whether a lethal injection is given. It also may be based on the physician's intent to hasten death, which is subjective and never absolutely knowable.[25] Reasonable observers might differ in their categorization of terminal sedation in terms of intent.[26] Similarly, what begins as voluntarily stopping eating and drinking in an alert, capable patient may become withholding life support from an incompetent patient as obtundation occurs. If the patient subsequently becomes delirious in this terminal phase, this practice might have to be followed by terminal sedation. Experienced clinicians could easily think of other complex examples in which the healthcare team and the family might be very challenged to find an adequate approach.

Each of these interventions, alone or in combination, may have a small place in end-of-life care for severely ill patients in whom the usual palliative treatments are failing. Only in the standard pain management case was death clearly unintended by both patient and physician—the risk of death was understood given the patient's grave condition, but it was not the goal of either party. Death was sought by the patient who stopped dexamethasone therapy, but it was not a certainty. With the other three interventions, death was the inevitable outcome and was actually sought by the patients. Although the physician's purpose in participating in these alternatives is to respond to human suffering, the decision-making process should include acknowledgment that death is inevitable. In any and all of these interventions, the physician must ensure the adequacy of palliative care and a full exploration of alternatives, the patient's mental capacity, and the proportionate presence of suffering.

Standard pain management and stopping life-sustaining therapy are standards of care, and all clinicians should be willing to provide these options. Even though voluntarily stopping eating and drinking and terminal sedation are legal, they are more extraordinary options, considered only when no acceptable alternatives are available and both patient and physician consider participation to be moral. Physician-assisted suicide remains illegal in most states. It should be exceedingly rare and provided only on request from the terminally ill patient whose suffering is intolerable and only when other alternatives are inadequate or incompatible with the patient's fundamental values. When physicians unilaterally choose not to participate in these options, they are obligated to search for acceptable alternatives with the patient. Ethics and palliative care consults may be helpful. If a mutually acceptable approach cannot be found, the patient and family should be given the option of transferring care to another physician.

NOTES

1. Council on Scientific Affairs, "Good care of the dying patient," *JAMA* 275 (1996): 474–78; American Board of Internal Medicine End-of-Life Patient Care Project Committee, *Caring for the Dying: Identification and Promotion of Physician Competency* (Philadelphia: American Board of Internal Medicine, 1996); Council on Ethical and Judicial Affairs, "Decisions near the end of life," *JAMA* 267 (1992): 2229–33; M. J. Field and C. K. Cassel eds., *Approaching Death: Improving Care at the End of Life* (Washington, D.C.: National Academy Press, 1997); K. M. Foley, "Pain, physician-assisted suicide, and euthanasia," *Pain Forum* 4 (1995): 163–78; T. E. Quill, *Death and Dignity: Making Choices and Taking Charge* (New York: W. W. Norton, 1993).

2. T. E. Quill, B. Lo, and D. W. Brock, "Palliative options of last resort: A comparison of voluntarily stoping eating and drinking, terminal sedation, physician-assisted suicide, and voluntary active euthanasia," *JAMA* 278 (1997): 2099–104.

3. See note 1.

4. L. H. Glantz, "Withholding and withdrawing treatment: The role of the criminal law," *Law Med Health Care* 15 (1987–88): 231–41; A. Meisel, "Legal myths about terminating life support," *Arch Intern Med* 151 (1991): 1497–502; D. K. Miller, R. M. Coe, and T. M. Hyers, "Achieving consensus on withdrawing or withholding care for critically ill patients," *J Gen Intern Med* 7 (1992): 475–80; H. Brody et al., "Withdrawing intensive life-sustaining treatment—recommendations for compassionate clinical management," *N Engl J Med* 336 (1997): 652–57; R. F. Weir and L. Gostin, "Decisions to abate life-sustaining treatment for nonautonomous patients: Ethical standards and legal liability for physicians after Cruzan," *JAMA* 264 (1990): 1846–53; W. C. Wilson et al., "Ordering and administration of sedatives and analgesics during the withholding and withdrawal of life support from critically ill patients," *JAMA* 267 (1992): 949–53.

5. Quill, Lo, and Brock, "Palliative options of last resort," pp. 2099–2104; R. D. Troug et al., "Barbiturates in the care of the terminally ill," *N Engl J Med* 327 (1991): 1678–82; N. I. Cherny and R. K. Portenoy, "Sedation in the management of refractory symptoms: Guidelines for evaluation and treatment," *J Palliat Care* 10 (1994): 31–38; V. Ventifridda et

al., "Symptom prevalence and control during cancer patients' last days of life," *J Palliat Care* 6 (1990): 7–11; J. L. Bernat, B. Gert, and R. P. Mogielnicki, "Patient refusal of hydration and nutrition: An alternative to physician-assisted suicide or voluntary active euthanasia," *Arch Intern Med* 153 (1993): 2723–28; L. A. Printz, "Terminal dehydration, a compassionate treatment," *Arch Intern Med* 153 (1992): 697–700; F. G. Miller and D. E. Meier, "Voluntary death: A comparison of terminal dehydration and physician-assisted suicide," *Ann Intern Med* 128 (1998): 559–62; T. E. Quill, "The ambiguity of clinical intentions," *N Engl J Med* 329 (1993): 1039–40; T. E. Quill, R. Dresser, and D. W. Brock, "The rule of double effect—a critique of its role in end-of-life decision making," *N Engl J Med* 337 (1997): 1768–71.

6. A. Alpers and B. Lo, "Physician-assisted suicide in Oregon: A bold experiment," *JAMA* 274 (1995): 483–87; A. E. Chin et al., "Legalized physician-assisted suicide in Oregon: the first year's experience," *N Engl J Med* 340 (1999): 577–83.

7. A. L. Back et al., "Physician-assisted suicide and euthanasia in Washington State: Patient requests and physician responses," *JAMA* 275 (1996): 919–25; D. Meier et al., "A national survey of physician-assisted suicide and euthanasia in the United States," *N Engl J Med* 338 (1998): 1193–1201.

8. Quill, Lo, and Brock, "Palliative options of last resort," pp. 2099–2104.

9. T. E. Quill, "Doctor, I want to die. Will you help me?" *JAMA* 270 (1993): 870–73; S. D. Block and J. A. Billings, "Patient requests to hasten death: Evaluation and management in terminal care," *Arch Intern Med* 154 (1994): 2039–47; F. Ackerman, "The significance of a wish," *Hastings Center Report* 21 (1991): 27–29; M. A. Rie, "The limits of a wish," *Hastings Center Report* 21 (1991): 24–27.

10. Alpers and Lo, "Physician-assisted suicide in Oregon," pp. 483–87. Chin et al., "Legalized physician-assisted suicide in Oregon," pp. 577–83.

11. Quill, Lo, and Brock, "Palliative options of last resort," pp. 2099–2104.

12. See note 1; also Quill, Lo, and Brock, "Palliative options of last resort," pp. 2099–2104.

13. T. E. Quill, "Principle of double effect and end-of-life pain man-

agement: Additional myths and a limited role," *J Palliat Med* 1 (1998): 333–36.

14. Quill, Dresser, and Brock, "The rule of double effect," pp. 1768–71.

15. See note 4.

16. Weir and Gostin, "Decisions to abate life-sustaining treatment," pp. 1846–53.

17. D. M. Eddy, "A piece of my mind: A conversation with my mother," *JAMA* 272 (1994): 179–81.

18. R. M. McCann, W. J. Hall, and A. Groth-Juncker, "Comfort care for terminally ill patients: The appropriate use of nutrition and hydration," *JAMA* 272 (1994): 1263–66.

19. Quill, Lo, and Brock, "Palliative options of last resort," pp. 2099–2104; Bernat, Gert, and Mogielnicki, "Patient refusal of hydration and nutrition," pp. 2723–28; Printz, "Terminal dehydration, a compassionate treatment," pp. 697–700; Miller and Meier, "Voluntary death," pp. 559–62.

20. Quill, Lo, and Brock, "Palliative options of last resort," pp. 2099–2104; Troug et al., "Barbiturates in the care of the terminally ill," pp. 1678–82; Cherny and Portenoy, "Sedation in the management of refractory symptoms," pp. 31–38; Ventifridda et al., "Symptom prevalence and control during cancer patients' last days of life," pp. 7–11.

21. Quill, Lo, and Brock, "Palliative options of last resort," pp. 2099–2104; Quill, "The ambiguity of clinical intentions," pp. 1039–40; Quill, Dresser, and Brock, "The rule of double effect," pp. 1768–71; J. A. Billings and S. D. Block, "Slow euthanasia," *J Palliat Care* 9 (1993): 21–30.

22. I. R. Byock, "Consciously walking the fine line: Thoughts on a hospice response to assisted suicide and euthanasia," *J Palliat Care* 9 (1993): 25–28; J. Lynn et al., "American geriatrics society on physician-assisted suicide: Brief to the United States Supreme Court," *J Am Geriatr Soc* 45 (1991): 691–94.

23. Cherny and Portenoy, "Sedation in the management of refractory symptoms," pp. 31–38.

24. Quill, *Death and Dignity*; Quill, Lo, and Brock, "Palliative options of last resort," pp. 2099–2104; Alpers and Lo, "Physician-assisted suicide in Oregon," pp. 483–87; Chin et al., "Legalized physician-assisted suicide in Oregon," pp. 577–83; Back et al., "Physician-assisted suicide and euthanasia in Washington State," pp. 919–25; Meier et al., "A national

survey of physician-assisted suicide and euthanasia in the United States," pp. 1193–1201; T. E. Quill, "Death and dignity: A case of individualized decision making," *N Engl J Med* 324 (1991): 691–94; T. E. Quill, C. K. Cassel, and D. E. Meier, "Care of the hopelessly ill: Proposed clinical criteria for physician-assisted suicide," *N Engl J Med* 327 (1997): 1380–84; S. H. Wanzer et al., "The physician's responsibility toward hopelessly ill patients: a second look," *N Engl J Med* 320 (1989): 844–49.

25. Quill, "The ambiguity of clinical intentions," pp. 1039–40; Quill, Dresser, and Brock, "The rule of double effect," pp. 1768–71.

26. Quill, Lo, and Brock, "Palliative options of last resort," pp. 2099–2104; Billings and Block, "Slow euthanasia," pp. 21–30.

8

CARING FOR THE DYING
Congressional Mischief

Marcia Angell

$\mathbf{F}$ive years ago, the citizens of Oregon voted by a narrow margin to legalize physician-assisted suicide for certain terminally ill patients. There followed a variety of efforts to nullify the decision, which culminated in a second referendum in 1997. This time Oregonians voted overwhelmingly to affirm their original decision, and Oregon is now the only state in which physician-assisted suicide is practiced legally.[1] Surveys indicate that most Americans and their doctors believe it should be available in all states.[2]

Shortly before the second Oregon vote, the U.S. Supreme Court considered the issue of physician-assisted suicide. The cases before it concerned state laws in Washington and New York that prohibit the practice. Opponents of those laws argued that they violated an implied constitutional right to choose, within limits, the time and manner of one's death—a right that would be unduly restricted if doctors were prohibited from helping.[3] The Court rejected that argument, unanimously finding no constitutional right to physician-assisted suicide.[4] However, it explicitly left the states free to legalize the practice through legislation or referendums, as in Oregon. Justice Sandra Day O'Connor, for example, referred warmly in her separate opinion to the serious work being done on this issue in the "laboratory of the states."

The Oregon law has now been in effect [since 1997]. Called the Death with Dignity Act, it permits physicians to prescribe a lethal dose of a controlled substance (usually a barbiturate) under well-defined circumstances. Patients may take the drug if and when they choose, but physicians may not themselves administer it. Initially, Oregon doctors were intimidated when the Drug Enforcement Administration warned that doctors who took part in physician-assisted suicide were violating the Controlled Substances Act and might lose their licenses to prescribe such drugs.[5] In June 1998, however, Attorney General Janet Reno put that fear to rest by stating that using controlled substances for physician-assisted suicide in accordance with Oregon law would not violate federal drug laws.

[In February 1998], the Oregon Health Division reported on the first year's experience with the new law.[6] It could find no evidence that the law had been abused. All told, fifteen Oregonians (thirteen with metastatic cancer, one with chronic obstructive pulmonary disease, and one with heart failure) chose to end their lives under the law's terms. Early indications are that the second year's experience will be similar.[7] This is hardly the carnage opponents predicted. But the availability of physician-assisted suicide may well have been a solace for many other terminally ill patients who ultimately decided not to make use of it. Furthermore, the intense public debate over the issue led Oregon to redouble its attention to all aspects of care at the end of life. The state now is widely acknowledged to offer some of the best palliative care in the country, and of course, the better the palliative care, the less likely patients are to choose physician-assisted suicide.

Despite the apparent successes of the Oregon law, another effort has been launched to thwart it, this time in the U.S. Congress. If successful, that effort will have pernicious consequences, not just for terminally ill patients in Oregon who would like the option of physician-assisted suicide, but also for dying patients throughout the country who merely want their last days to be comfortable. Once again, the tool being used is the Controlled Substances Act. On October 27, 1999, the House of Representatives voted to amend the act to make it a federal crime, punishable by twenty years in prison, for doctors to prescribe drugs for terminally ill patients to end their lives.[8] The Senate is now considering the same bill. Called the Pain Relief Promotion Act of 1999, the bill's purpose is "to amend the Controlled Substances Act to promote pain management and palliative care without permitting assisted suicide and euthanasia, and for other purposes."[9] It states that the attorney general "shall give no force and effect to state law authorizing or permitting assisted suicide or euthanasia," thus overriding Reno's earlier decision to defer to the voters of Oregon.

That may seem a small price to pay if the bill really promotes better pain relief, as its title promises. But the title is misleading. If the bill becomes law, it will almost certainly discourage doctors from prescribing or administering adequate doses of drugs to relieve the symptoms of dying patients. To be sure, the bill pays lip service to promoting adequate pain relief. It states that doctors may use controlled substances to alleviate pain or discomfort, "even if the use of such a substance may increase the risk of death" —a prerogative doctors have always had. But in the next sentence, it forbids "intentionally dispensing, distributing, or administering a controlled substance for the purpose of causing death or assisting another person in causing death." Thus, the bill turns on discerning physicians' intentions in administering controlled substances and provides for harsh penalties if those intentions are found not to conform with a "legitimate medical purpose."

The bill's effects would be felt more by terminally ill patients who do not wish physician-assisted suicide than by those who do, since there are so many more of them. Many terminally ill patients require extremely high doses of controlled substances for adequate relief of symptoms. Doctors, faced with the possibility of long prison sentences if their intentions are misread, may be reluctant to prescribe or administer such doses. Treatment of pain in the terminally ill is already notoriously inadequate, largely because our society's preoccupation with drug abuse seeps into the medical arena. Many doctors are concerned about the scrutiny they invite when they prescribe or administer controlled substances, and they are hypersensitive to "drug-seeking behavior" in patients. Patients, as well as doctors, often have exaggerated fears of addiction and the side effects of narcotics. Congress would make this bad situation worse.

Furthermore, when the suffering of a dying patient is prolonged and intractable, a doctor who administers or prescribes large doses of a controlled substance may well have mixed intentions. Just as family members often feel a sense of relief along with their grief when such patients finally die, so doctors often wish both to ease suffering and to hasten death. The balance of those desires may vary from hour to hour, depending on the patient's condition. The congressional bill holds that it is permissible to hasten death only if that is not the intent. That view, which is based on a thirteenth-century theological argument called the "doctrine of double effect," is too simplistic to capture the mixed feelings of doctors who are caring for grievously suffering patients. If all attempts at palliation fail, as they sometimes do, then the hope for an easier death may give way to the hope for a faster one. That is, the intent can shift.

Intent matters in criminal law. For example, whether a motorist who runs someone down is charged with homicide or manslaughter depends on whether it was done deliberately. The motorist knows what the intent was, even if it is difficult to prove in court, and whatever the intent, no one—least of all the victim—could approve of the act. But the situation is different for compassionate doctors caring for the terminally ill. They simply want to relieve their patients' suffering, and that is what their patients want and expect of them, sometimes in whatever way possible. Not only is it difficult in such cases to parse the intent behind each element in the treatment, it is also doubtful that anyone should want to try. Mercy, especially in doctors, is not something to be rooted out. That is why the application of criminal law is inappropriate in this setting. It is absurd to imagine that doctors could be innocent in one hour, but deserving of twenty years in prison in the next, simply because the desired outcome of treatment changed. What is important is whether doctors are doing their utmost to ease suffering in accord with their patients' wishes.

Opposition to the bill comes not just from those who are concerned about adequate relief of symptoms for the terminally ill or from those who favor legalizing physician-assisted suicide. It also comes from those who see the bill as a meddlesome encroachment on the practice of medicine. Many doctors believe that the authors of the bill, in defining legitimate medical use, are assuming the prerogatives of the medical profession. Not surprisingly, medical associations are divided on the issue. The American Medical Association, which opposes physician-assisted suicide, supports the bill. The Massachusetts Medical Society, which also opposes physician-assisted suicide, has attacked the bill as an unwarranted intrusion into medical practice that would have "a chilling effect on prescribing adequate medicine."[10]

In addition, proponents of states' rights are dismayed by the attempt of the bill's supporters to thwart Oregon's law by misusing Congress's authority to regulate drugs. The Controlled Substances Act was enacted in 1970 to prevent and control drug abuse, not to define the medical uses of drugs.[11] The aim was to interrupt the flow of illicit drugs to the streets. The congressional bill is now seizing on a stratagem far removed from the act's original purpose simply to nullify Oregon's law. Ironically, the principal supporters of the bill are conservative Republicans, ostensibly committed to both individual liberty and states' rights. Yet they would restrict the liberty of dying patients and the rights of states to regulate the practice of medicine.

If the bill passes both houses of Congress and is signed into law by the president, Oregon will probably challenge the law in the courts. Even many Oregonians who opposed physician-assisted suicide in the state referendums, including the Oregon Medical Association, resent the attempt by Congress to overturn the outcome.[12] The case might then reach the Supreme Court. If it does, one can hope that the justices will remember their commitment to the laboratory of the states. Otherwise, Congress will have done great harm—to dying patients, both those who want the option of physician-assisted suicide and those who simply want their suffering relieved, and to their physicians, who should be able to offer compassionate care without fear of reprisal.

NOTES

1. Oregon Death with Dignity Act, Oregon Revised Statute 127.800127.897.

2. R. J. Blendon, U. S. Szalay, and R. A. Knox, "Should physicians aid their patients in dying? The public perspective," *JAMA* 267 (1992): 2658–62; J. G. Bachman et al., "Attitudes of Michigan physicians and the public toward legalizing physician-assisted suicide and voluntary euthanasia, *N Engl J Med* 334 (1996): 303–309; M. A. Lee et al., "Legalizing assisted suicide—views of physicians in Oregon," *N Engl J Med* 334 (1996): 310–15.

3. M. Angell, "The Supreme Court and physician-assisted suicide—the ultimate right," *N Engl J Med* 336 (1997): 50–53.

4. *Vacco* v. *Quill*, U.S. Supreme Court, 95-1858 (26 June 1997); *Washington* v. *Glucksberg*, U.S. Supreme Court, 96-110 (26 June 1997).

5. "Threat from Washington has chilling effect on Oregon law allowing assisted suicide," *New York Times*, 19 November 1997, A16.

6. A. E. Chin et al., "Legalized physician-assisted suicide in Oregon —the first year's experience," *N Engl J Med* 340 (1999): 577–83.

7. K. Hedberg, personal communication.

8. "House backs ban on using medicine to aid in suicide," *New York Times*, 28 October 1999, A1; A. E. Kornblut, "Ban on prescribing drugs for suicide gets House OK," *Boston Globe*, 28 October 1999, A1.

9. *Pain Relief Promotion Act of 1999*, 106th Congress, 1st session, H.R. 2260.

10. Kornblut, "Ban on prescribing drugs for suicide gets House OK."

11. *Controlled Substances Act of 1970*, 21 USC Sec. 823.

12. S. H. Verhovek, "Oregon chafes at measure to stop assisted suicides," *New York Times*, 28 October 1999, A1.

9

HOUSE TESTIMONY ON THE PAIN RELIEF PROMOTION ACT OF 1999

Ann Jackson

My name is Ann Jackson. I am the executive director and chief executive officer of the Oregon Hospice Association (OHA). OHA is a 501(c)(3) public benefit organization dedicated to ensuring that all Oregonians have access to high-quality hospice and comfort care. It has established expertise concerning all end-of-life options in Oregon.

OHA and Oregon's hospice providers are very concerned that the Pain Relief Promotion Act of 1999, like the Lethal Drug Abuse Prevention Act of 1998, will have a negative impact on pain and symptom management throughout the healthcare continuum in Oregon and throughout the country. OHA opposes the Pain Relief Promotion Act of 1999.

I am a member of the Task Force to Improve Care of Terminally Ill Oregonians, a consortium of twenty-four individuals who represent state healthcare professional organizations, state agencies

House Committee on the Judiciary, Subcommittee on the Constitution, *The Pain Relief Promotion Act of 1999: Hearing on H.R. 2260,* written testimony of Ann Jackson, M.M., June 24, 1999.

involved with healthcare, and health systems in the Portland metropolitan area. The task force, which remains neutral on physician-assisted suicide, was convened in December, 1994. Its purpose is to promote excellent care of the dying and to address the ethical and clinical issues posed by the enactment of the Death with Dignity Act. The task force has published two documents: (1) *The Final Months of Life: A Guide to Oregon Resources;* and (2) *The Oregon Death with Dignity Act: A Guidebook for Health Care Providers.*

The Task Force to Improve Care of Terminally Ill Oregonians is concerned that the Pain Relief Promotion Act of 1999 will have a negative impact on pain and symptom management at the end of life.[1]

I am here today representing both OHA and the Task Force to Improve Care of Terminally Ill Oregonians. Neither group believes it possible that a law that will increase regulatory scrutiny and judge the "intent" of all healthcare providers can promote pain relief. Both groups are also concerned about the potential long-term negative impact that may result from restrictively defining palliative care, and drawing too narrow a line between appropriate and inappropriate uses of controlled substances.

I am also a member of the Physician Orders for Life-Sustaining Treatment Task Force (POLST), whose goal is to ensure that Oregonians' end-of-life wishes are respected. The POLST form translates advance directives into doctors' orders.[2] I am active, too, in the Health Ethics Network of Oregon.

Finally, OHA is represented on Oregon's Legislative Task Force on Pain and Symptom Management. During the past two years I have both testified on behalf of OHA and represented OHA on the task force at regional meetings, identifying barriers to pain management. Unrelieved pain—terminal pain, chronic pain, cancer pain, postsurgical pain—is epidemic throughout the country. Even in Oregon where the Board of Medical Examiners has urged physicians to address pain and other symptoms aggressively. Even in Oregon, which is recognized as the national leader in end-of-life care.[3]

REGULATORY SCRUTINY CAUSES A CHILLING EFFECT ON PHYSICIAN PRESCRIBING PRACTICES

At every meeting of the Task Force on Pain and Symptom Management, a parade of physicians testified that regulatory scrutiny was the cause of the unrelieved pain problem. Even the threat of an investigation has a chilling effect on prescribing practices, regardless of whether that threat comes from the DEA, the Board of Medical Examiners, or the local coroner, and regardless of whether that threat is real or perceived. This is not an unusual response for law-abiding citizens: when most Americans encounter a police car parked at the side of the highway, they slow down *below* the posted speed. This is not to suggest that no rules should apply to healthcare workers. It is, however, meant to say that the climate that already exists in end-of-life care encourages levels of caution which too frequently result in increased pain and suffering for sick and dying people. This proposed bill would only worsen those conditions.

ATTEMPTS TO MEASURE INTENT WILL CAUSE A CHILLING EFFECT ON PHYSICIAN PRESCRIBING PRACTICES

While others are comforted that a medical advisory board is not included in the proposed 1999 legislation, we remain alarmed. We believe that this year's provision for the education and training of state, local, and federal law enforcement personnel in the appropriate use of controlled substances is an even more hazardous substitute. It is unrealistic to think the secretary of health and human services will be more successful at effectively training law enforcement officials than medical schools or boards of medical examiners have been at training physicians. If this bill is passed, the standard of care for any community will be determined by the investigative judgment or whim of its local law enforcement personnel. Rather than one unified standard across the states, there will be many, often conflicting standards, even within each state.

A NARROW DEFINITION OF PALLIATIVE CARE WILL CAUSE A CHILLING EFFECT ON PHYSICIAN PRESCRIBING PRACTICES

While we applaud efforts to establish that controlled substances should be used for pain control, even if the use of such substances may increase the likelihood of death, the bill's definition of palliative care negates that provision when it codifies into law ambiguous goals. Palliative care *seeks* to neither hasten nor postpone death. But it would be inhumane to not palliate inevitable pain and other symptoms of a patient who has asked to be removed from a ventilator, when her intent is to hasten her death. It would be inhumane to deny a patient interventions that may postpone death just long enough to reach an important milestone, such as the wedding of a cherished daughter. Hastening or postponing the dying process, while not usual, does happen under good palliative care. While palliative care is an evolving specialty, it is so narrowly defined in this bill that the effect will be to put its practitioners into a too rigid box.

A NARROW LINE DRAWING THE DISTINCTION BETWEEN APPROPRIATE AND INAPPROPRIATE USES OF CONTROLLED SUBSTANCES WILL CAUSE A CHILLING EFFECT ON PHYSICIAN PRESCRIBING PRACTICES

A goal of the Pain Relief Promotion Act is to make a clear distinction between an appropriate use of controlled substances to manage pain, even if death is hastened inadvertently, and an inappropriate use of controlled substances to assist in a suicide. It attempts to make black and white a very gray area, creating a tightrope, when a balance beam or even a bench would be both more acceptable and defensible. The use of controlled substances is always subject to question, when our society has invested so much time to curb their abuse. Questions will be raised by pharmacists, nurses, health aides, or family members, any of whom may be alarmed by what they perceive to be unusually large doses of narcotics or other drugs—or a death following soon on the heels of a prescription. These questions will precipitate an investigation. These investigations will significantly undermine physicians' prescribing practices.

And it will be America's rural communities that suffer most. Rural physicians are often subject to more scrutiny. Urban physicians have more ready access to the latest information concerning pain management. Urban physicians have better access to pain specialists. Therefore urban physicians are more confident in their ability to defend their use of a controlled substance.

Regardless of its "intent," by trying to draw a clear line, the Pain Relief Promotion Act will prompt frequent questioning of the intent to manage pain versus the intent to cause death. It's very safe to say that every hospice in the country has had a request for help to die from at least one of its patients, not just Oregon hospices. Are those patients no longer entitled to have their symptoms relieved because they voiced that desire, because someone may question whether the intent of the physician was to grant their request or to relieve their symptoms?

CONCLUSION

When Senator Nickles introduced the Pain Relief Promotion Act in the Senate, he indicated that a dynamic was created whereby some doctors underutilized controlled substances for pain. Hospices report that such instances were isolated and, most often, readily corrected. It was not until November, 1997, when the DEA issued its letter indicating that it would prosecute physicians who prescribed controlled substances under the Death with Dignity Act, that we saw a downward turn in what had been a steady increase in the use of controlled substances for pain and symptom management in Oregon. While we do not know that the letter from Mr. Constantine was the cause, the timing is suspicious. Copies of the Fall 1998 Oregon BME Newsletter documenting this trend have been made available to the subcommittee.[4]

OHA and the Task Force to Improve Care of Terminally Ill Oregonians have grave concerns about the Pain Relief Promotion Act of 1999. We are strongly convinced that this legislation, if passed, will have a profoundly negative impact on physician prescribing practices all across the United States. We are as strongly committed as we were last year that this law be challenged and defeated.

The Conquering Pain Act and the Advance Planning and Compassionate Care Act are more likely to accomplish much needed improvement in end-of-life care than the Pain Relief Promotion Act of 1999. Efforts to reduce unwarranted, unnecessary, and excessive regulatory scrutiny of the nation's hospices will accomplish improvement in end-of-life care. Efforts to reduce futile care will accomplish improvement in end-of-life care. The Pain Relief Promotion Act will not.

NOTES

1. A statement and list of task force members was made available to the subcommittee.

2. "Focus: Oregon's POLST program," *State Initiatives in End-of-Life Care*, no. 3 (April 1999).

3. "Focus: Oregon," *State Initiatives in End-of-Life Care*, no. 1 (June 1998).

4. S. Tolle and K. Haley, "Pain management in the dying, successes and concerns," *Oregon BME Newsletter* (fall 1998).

1 0

HOUSE TESTIMONY ON THE PAIN RELIEF PROMOTION ACT OF 1999

N. Gregory Hamilton for Physicians for Compassionate Care

SUMMARY STATEMENT

Physicians for Compassionate Care, an organization providing education about pain relief and palliative care, urges passage of the Pain Relief Promotion Act of 1999. The need for education on state-of-the-art pain management and palliative care is overwhelming. Individual medical organizations cannot do it alone. A nationwide and federally sponsored educational effort is required. This proposed legislation goes a long way toward helping doctors and nurses meet the needs of suffering patients.

The Pain Relief Promotion Act clarifies to law enforcement officers, as well as to physicians, nurses, and state medical boards, that provision of pain medicine is a legitimate medical practice, even if in rare instances there may be an added risk to a patient's life. That clarification will reassure doctors, nurses, and hospice

House Committee on the Judiciary, Subcommittee on the Constitution, *The Pain Relief Promotion Act of 1999: Hearing on H.R. 2260,* testimony of N. Gregory Hamilton for Physicians for Compassionate Care, June 24, 1999.

workers that they need not fear while providing patients necessary care. Equally important, this legislation reconfirms that controlled substances may not be used intentionally to kill patients in any of the fifty states, as is currently the case in forty-nine states.

Assisted suicide and euthanasia inevitably interfere with pain management and palliative care. In Oregon, its rationed health plan for the poor denies payment for 171 needed services while it fully funds assisted suicide. More than 38 percent of Oregon Health Plan members report barriers to obtaining mental health services, yet assisted suicide costs the state as little as forty-five dollars, according to its own estimates. Oregon insurance companies and health maintenance organizations (HMOs) generally limit benefits to two key elements of palliative care—mental health and hospice care benefits. One Oregon HMO (Qual Med) caps in-home palliative care (hospice) at one thousand dollars while fully funding assisted suicide. Education of professionals and clarification that killing patients is not legitimate medical treatment will go a long way to assure improved care at the end of life.

Physicians for Compassionate Care urges passage of the Pain Relief Promotion Act of 1999 to protect patients and their doctors.

At each of Physicians for Compassionate Care's last two advanced pain and palliative care conferences, national experts told our audiences that they could reassure their patients they do not need to die in unrelieved pain. Then, they proceeded to teach cancer doctors and nurses, hospice workers and psychiatrists, anesthesiologists and pain specialists state-of-the-art techniques available to make such a claim supportable.

Treatments for pain and other elements of suffering have improved dramatically over the past twenty years in the United States. Yet many, perhaps most, physicians and other health professionals remain unaware of the high success rate of recent advances in the use of pain-relieving drug regimens and procedures for control of severe pain in the seriously ill.

Conferences by voluntary organizations such as ours, however, cannot, by themselves, fill the gap between available treatments and knowledge of those treatments. Our Compassionate Care Conference will be joined by two additional conferences on palliative care of the seriously ill in the state of Oregon this fall. Yet the few hundred participants in these conferences pale by comparison to the more than eight thousand physicians practicing in our small state alone, in addition to the thousands of nurses and hospice workers. Nationwide, the magnitude of the problem is staggering. Even broad-ranging educational programs, such as those developed by the American Medical Association, are not enough. There is still woefully inadequate pain care training of most physicians. A national, coordinated, and funded effort is required to provide clinicians with the needed skills to alleviate the suffering of those ailing in our society. The Pain Relief Promotion Act goes a long way to provide the educational and research resources required to meet the physical, psychological, social, and spiritual needs of suffering individuals.

AGGRESSIVE PAIN MANAGEMENT IS LEGITIMATE

The Pain Relief Promotion Act wisely emphasizes that aggressive pain management is a legitimate medical use of controlled substances, even if, in rare circumstances, such treatment may increase the risk of death. This reassurance is entirely compatible with the long-standing ethics and practices of virtually all medical organizations, including the American Medical Association. In the vast majority of cases, it is fairly easy, given some degree of prudence, to ascertain that aggressive pain care will not kill the patient. It usually takes manyfold the dose of an opioid to suppress respiration than it takes to alleviate pain or cause drowsiness, and there is medication available to reverse rapidly an inadvertent excessive dose of such medicines. Nevertheless, rarely and under extreme circumstances, pain medicines can pose some unwanted risk to life. This bill protects physicians, nurses, and patients in the event of such a circumstance.

Some proponents of assisted suicide have tried to portray this time-honored distinction between a rare, unintended death and intentional euthanasia or assisted suicide as arbitrary or disingenuous. Nothing could be farther from the truth. Both doctors and patients historically have relied upon the clarity of the doctor's intention to comfort but never kill as a guiding principle. Religion and the law have adopted the same principle. In 1997, the United States Supreme Court reaffirmed that intent is a valid and verifiable legal concept. It declared in *Vacco* v. *Quill et al.* that ". . . in some cases, pain killing drugs may hasten a patient's death, but the physician's purpose and intent is, or may be, only to ease his patient's pain." A doctor who assists a suicide, however, "must necessarily and indubitably intend primarily that the patient be made dead." The Supreme Court went on to emphasize that "the law has long used doctors' intent or purpose to distinguish between two acts that may have the same result." The distinction is clear enough. It is not possible to write a prescription for ninety barbiturates to be taken all at once, as has been the case in nearly all Oregon assisted suicides, without intending to kill the patient. In such a case, the intent is clear. Fortunately, most doctors have no such intention and do not prescribe ninety barbiturates to be taken at once, or twenty to fifty times the patient's most recent morphine dose to be injected quickly. The intention of the vast majority of doctors in prescribing pain medicine is clear enough, also. It is to alleviate suffering but never to kill. The Pain Relief Prevention Act makes this distinction clearly. It thereby protects doctors from inadvertent prosecution, even investigation, in all fifty states.

Apparent attempts by some to obscure this distinction make the need to educate law enforcement personnel, as well as health professionals, all the more pressing. The Pain Relief Promotion Act provides for the education of both law enforcement personnel and regulatory bodies.

Some public safety dangers inherent in leaving unclear the distinction between legitimate medical procedures and assisted suicide, as does the June 5, 1998, opinion of U.S. Attorney General Janet Reno, have been outlined in previous testimony before this subcommittee on July 14, 1998.

11

EXISTENTIAL SUFFERING AND PALLIATIVE SEDATION
A Brief Commentary with a Proposal for Clinical Guidelines

Paul Rousseau

Palliative sedation (PS) is a valuable and contentious intervention that is utilized to manage refractory symptoms in terminal illness, and was fundamentally sanctioned by the United States Supreme Court in its 1997 decision negating a constitutional right to physician-assisted suicide.[1] Although not a frequent palliative intervention, the incidence of PS varies from 2 percent to 52 percent, with such variance attributable to diverse definitions of PS,[2] the retrospective nature of studies, and cultural, religious, and ethnic disparities.[3]

While the definition of PS can be subjective and ambiguous, many clinicians define it as the act of purposely inducing and maintaining a pharmacologically sedated and unconscious state, without the intent to cause death, in select circumstances complicated by refractory symptoms.[4] Similar to PS, the definition of a refractory symptom can likewise be subjective and ambiguous;

Reprinted from *American Journal of Hospice & Palliative Care* 18, no. 3 (May/June 2001): 151–53.

however, Cherny and Portenoy provide a clinically acceptable explication of a refractory symptom as one that cannot be adequately controlled despite aggressive efforts to identify a tolerable therapy that does not compromise consciousness. They further add that a symptom may be considered refractory when additional invasive and noninvasive interventions are incapable of providing adequate relief, or the therapy is associated with excessive and intolerable acute or chronic morbidity and is unlikely to provide relief within an acceptable time frame.[5] While sedation for refractory physical symptoms may be more readily accepted by clinicians, patients, and families, existential suffering can be just as refractory and agonizing as physical symptoms. However, Cherny notes that unlike refractory physical symptoms, there are no well-established strategies for evaluating and managing refractory existential distress.[6] For instance, the various tumors and their associated symptoms and standard therapies are well known and documented, whereas no simple and clinically oriented evaluative and therapeutic method exists for the many spiritual and psychosocial concerns encompassing existential suffering. In addition, PS for existential symptoms can be emotionally, ethically, and morally challenging for healthcare providers and family, as the patient is frequently awake, cognitively intact, and socially interacting prior to initiation of sedation.[7] What's more, existential suffering may not be associated with significant physiological deterioration, further confounding many healthcare providers' clinical decision to use sedative therapy.[8] Accordingly, existential distress may be perceived by clinicians and families as an ethically and morally inappropriate indication for the utilization of PS. However, as astutely noted by Rosen, a medical model that assesses psychological or spiritual aspects of patients' lives as a function of physical condition is shortsighted and may even be harmful.[9] In the end, when the goal of care is patient comfort and relief of debilitating symptoms, sedation can be a useful palliative adjunct to mitigate the anguish of disabling existential suffering.

ETHICAL JUSTIFICATION

In the wake of the Supreme Court decision regarding physician-assisted suicide and the justices' seemingly "legal" approbation of PS, renewed interest and debate have arisen, with some contending that sedative therapy is nothing more than assisted suicide. Consequently, the ethics of this practice have been questioned, particularly where existential suffering and nutrition and hydration are involved.

Traditionally, the ethical justification for PS has been derived from the principle of double effect, a tenet developed by Roman Catholic theologians in the Middle Ages.[10] The doctrine of double effect succinctly emphasizes the intent of the clinician and incorporates four cardinal precepts: (1) the nature of the act must be good or morally neutral and not intrinsically wrong; (2) the intent of the clinician must be good, with the good effect and not the bad effect intended, although the bad effect can be foreseen and permitted; (3) the bad effect must not be the means to the good effect; and (4) there must be proportionality, in that the good effect must exceed or balance the bad effect.[11] Autonomy is an additional ethical principle that is valuable in the ethical and moral justification of sedative pharmacotherapy. Autonomy, defined as a patient's right to make independent and uncoerced decisions regarding treatment preferences, permits patients with decision-making capacity singularly to elect or reject medical therapy, based upon their personal moral, ethical, religious, and informed understanding of the benefits and burdens of treatment.[12] Such a decision is justifiable, irrespective of the clinician's medical, ethical, and moral judgment regarding the patient's choice, except in situations involving euthanasia and physician-assisted suicide (apart from Oregon, where a physician may provide assisted suicide to a competent, terminally ill patient). However, autonomy is clinically tempered by the fact that a clinician is not obliged to provide care that violates his or her values and morals. In such situations, care can and should be transferred to another provider willing to abide by the patient's request. The clinician must remain vigilant and cognizant that, in rare circumstances, patients may request PS with a surreptitious goal of hastened and intended death. In such cases, psychological or psychiatric consultations are obligatory in an effort to ascertain the origin and desire for a premature death, and attempt to alleviate the precipitants of a covert request for an impulsive death.

The ethical and moral dilemmas associated with terminating nutrition and hydration when instituting PS prompted Quill and associates to argue that patients often die of dehydration, starvation, or some other intervening complication, not the underlying disease, as promulgated by proponents of PS. In fact, Quill et al. argue that withholding nutrition and fluids is typically taken to hasten a patient's wished-for death.[13] However, many patients have already limited their oral intake, or completely stopped eating and drinking due to the anorexia of advanced disease; for that reason, the absence of nutrition and hydration is not necessarily a conduit to a patient's wished-for death, but rather a poorly understood physiologic reaction to chronic and debilitating disease. Moreover, many patients do not wish for death as espoused by Quill et al., but rather relief from daily suffering that at times is interminable and reduces any remaining quality of life. However, if intravenous or subcutaneous hydration is present, discussion must ensue regarding the benefits and burdens of hydration at the end of life, and, in particular, the futility of such therapy in a patient selecting PS. A similar discussion should be initiated with patients receiving enteral or total parenteral nutrition. In contemporary ethical, legal, and clinical discourse, nutrition and hydration are considered extraordinary care, and the ethical validity of discontinuing these interventions in a patient selecting PS is categorically based upon responsible ethical and legal judiciousness. All the same, PS and the withdrawal of nutrition and hydration remain controversial, as their use increases in hospice and palliative care programs.

PROPOSED CRITERIA FOR PALLIATIVE SEDATION OF EXISTENTIAL SUFFERING

As noted by Cherny, it is not desirable either to subject patients with refractory existential suffering to protracted trials of therapies that provide inadequate relief, or to sedate patients when viable alternatives remain.[14] In addition, refractory existential suffering must be distinguished from problematical issues that may respond to appropriate therapy, including depression, delirium, anxiety, and familial discord. To assist in decision making regarding PS in existential suffering, the following clinical guidelines are proposed: (1) the patient must have a terminal illness; (2) a do-not-resuscitate (DNR) order must be in effect; (3) all palliative treatments must be exhausted, including treatments for depression, delirium, anxiety, and any other contributing maladies;[15] (4) a psychological assessment by a skilled clinician should be completed; (5) an assessment for spiritual issues by a skilled clinician or clergy member should be completed; (6) if nutritional support or intravenous or subcutaneous hydration is present, discussion should be initiated regarding the benefits and burdens of such therapy in view of impending PS; (7) informed consent should be obtained from the patient or surrogate decision maker; and (8) consideration should be given to an initial trial of respite sedation.[16] The latter concept involves sedating the patient for a predetermined interval, such as twenty-four to forty-eight hours, then downwardly titrating the sedative until consciousness reappears. With respite sedation, second-guessing and reassessment by healthcare providers, patients, and family members may be accomplished,[17] but, more important, an indeterminate number of patients may break a cycle of anxiety and distress that precipitated the request for PS and nullify the need for further sedation.[18] If a trial of respite sedation is rejected in favor of continuous sedation, patients and families must be informed that it may take days or weeks before death occurs; such a time period can be emotionally chaotic for families and may precipitate second-guessing, psychological distress, and familial dissension. Support is crucial and must be provided during this time to both family members and healthcare staff.

Finally, once PS is initiated, the dosage of the sedative agent should not be increased unless the patient awakens, is restless or grimaces, withdraws from touch and other stimuli, or has any other findings that could reasonably be interpreted as evidence of suffering, including tachypnea or tachycardia. As noted by Alpers and Lo, increasing sedation without an overt clinical indication might imply the clinician is intending to hasten death and would ostensibly cross the line between PS and physician-assisted suicide or euthanasia.[19]

CONCLUSION

The dying process can be a time of growth, reconciliation, and spiritual enrichment; however, it can also be a time of considerable suffering, abolishing hope of a peaceful and tranquil death. The main goal of a physician is to relieve suffering, but when suffering becomes refractory to standard palliative therapies, PS offers a humane alternative to conscious and continual anguish. Although PS is more readily accepted as a palliative strategy in physical suffering, existential anguish can be equally debilitating and may warrant aggressive palliation. Consequently, in cases where existential suffering is unabated, PS offers an acceptable alternative to intractable existential distress.

NOTES

1. P. C. Rousseau, "Palliative sedation: A brief review of ethical validity and clinical experience," *Mayo Clinic Proc* 75 (2000): 1064–69; *Vacco* v. *Quill*, 117 S. Ct. 2293 (1997); *Washington* v. *Glucksberg*, 117 S. Ct. 2258 (1997).

2. Rousseau, "Palliative sedation," pp. 1064–69; T. E. Quill, R. Dresser, and D. W. Brock, "The rule of double effect—A critique of its role in end-of-life decision making," *N Engl J Med* 337 (1997): 1768–71.

3. Rousseau, "Palliative sedation," pp. 1064–69; R. L. Fainsinger et al., "Sedation for delirium and other symptoms in terminally ill patients in Edmonton," *J Palliat Care* 16 (2000): 5–10.

4. R. L. Fainsinger et al., "Sedation for uncontrolled symptoms in a South African hospice," *J Pain & Symp Mgmnt* 16 (1998): 145–52; J. Hallenbeck, "Terminal sedation for intractable distress: Not slow euthanasia but a prompt response to suffering," *West J Med* 171 (1999): 222–23; N. I. Cherny and R. K. Portenoy, "Sedation in the management of refractory symptoms: Guidelines for evaluation and treatment," *J Palliat Care* 10 (1994): 31–38.

5. Cherny and Portenoy, "Sedation in the management of refractory symptoms," pp. 31–38.

6. N. I. Cherny, "Sedation in response to refractory existential distress: Walking the fine line," *J Pain & Symp Mgmnt* 16 (1998): 406–407.

7. Rousseau, "Palliative sedation," pp. 1064–69.

8. Cherny, "Sedation in response to refractory existential distress: Walking the fine line," pp. 406–407.

9. E. J. Rosen, "A case of 'terminal sedation' in the family," *J Pain & Symp Mgmnt* 16 (1998): 406–407.

10. Quill, Dresser, and Brock, "The rule of double effect," pp. 1768–71; T. E. Quill, B. Lo, and D. W. Brock, "Palliative options of last resort: A comparison of voluntarily stopping eating and drinking, terminal sedation, physician-assisted suicide, and voluntary active euthanasia," *JAMA* 278 (1997): 2099–2104.

11. T. L. Beauchamp and J. F. Childress, *Principles of Biomedical Ethics* (New York: Oxford University Press, 1989).

12. P. C. Rousseau, "Ethical concepts in hospice and palliative medicine," in *Hospice and Palliative Medicine: Core Curriculum and Review Syllabus*, ed. R. S. Schonwetter, W. Hawke, and C. F. Knight (Dubuque, Iowa: Kendall/Hunt Publishing, 1999), pp. 153–58.

13. Quill, Lo, and Brock, "Palliative options of last resort," pp. 2099–2104.

14. Cherny, "Sedation in response to refractory existential distress: Walking the fine line," pp. 406–407.

15. Rousseau, "Ethical concepts in hospice and palliative medicine," pp. 153–58.

16. Cherny, "Sedation in response to refractory existential distress: Walking the fine line," pp. 406–407.

17. Rousseau, "Palliative sedation," pp. 1064–69; Quill, Lo, and Brock, "Palliative options of last resort," pp. 2099–2104.

18. Cherny, "Sedation in response to refractory existential distress: Walking the fine line," pp. 406–407.

19. A. Alpers and B. Lo, "The Supreme Court addresses physician-assisted suicide: Can its rulings improve palliative care?" *Arch Fam Med* 8 (1999): 200–205.

12

PALLIATIVE SEDATION vs. TERMINAL SEDATION
What's in a Name?

W. Clay Jackson

P aul Rousseau's recent discussions of existential suffering and proposal of clinical guidelines for the sedation of patients with intractable physical, mental, or spiritual distress"[1] are cogent, welcome contributions to the field of palliative medicine. His comments contain much to admire, including the emphasis on the patient's symptoms, not the patient's death, as the focus of care. His recommendation that the treatment (including drug dosages) be adjusted based on the patient's symptoms gives this sometimes controversial practice a sensible clinical platform that withstands rigorous ethical investigation (for example, utilizing Jonsen's four-box method[2] of clinical ethical analysis). Content notwithstanding, however, I most admire Rousseau's reviews for what they lack— the perpetuation of the linguistic quagmire, "terminal sedation."

Attributed to Robert E. Enck, M.D.,[3] the phrase *terminal sedation* is commonly used for the clinical practice of utilizing therapeutic sedation in imminently dying patients, as a means of palli-

Reprinted from *American Journal of Hospice & Palliative Care* 19, no. 2 (March/April 2002): 81–82.

ating symptoms which are not ameliorated by other, less aggressive measures. Debate concerning the ethical implications of the practice has been, at times, lively—ranging from case descriptions praising its efficacy and humaneness[4] to editorials decrying it as "slow euthanasia."[5] For most clinicians, however, the practice seems to be an acceptable method of treating patients with otherwise intractable symptoms, provided that the focus of drug titration is symptom relief, not the patient's death.[6] This distinction appeals to the ethical principle of double effect: if the patient's death is an undesired but anticipated secondary effect of the treatment, this is allowable, as the secondary effect was not intended.[7]

As this intervention grows in acceptance and in frequency, the use of the term *terminal sedation* to describe it should be abandoned. As Chatter et al. have pointed out,[8] the phrase is confusing, in that the object of the adjective "terminal" is not

explicit. Does it apply to the sedation (implying that the object of the practice is sedating someone to death) or to the patient (implying that the patient is in the final stage of illness)? Since this ambiguity is always present, the phrase is often interpreted to imply intent to kill. This interpretation has the potential to restrict patient access to state-of-the art palliative care, by leaving patients and families confused about their physicians' intent, and by leaving physicians fearful that their palliative interventions will be wrongly prejudged as "mercy killing."[9]

These considerations notwithstanding, many authors[10] (formerly including Rousseau himself)[11] have persisted in describing the clinical practice of sedating terminally ill patients with intractable physical, mental, or spiritual distress as terminal sedation. In explaining their position, Quill and Byock maintain that doing so is necessary to distinguish sedation in antemortem care from sedation in other settings (such as the treatment of burn victims), and to lend a sense of *gravitas* to the sedation of the terminally ill.[12] I find this explanation unconvincing, in that the context of palliative sedation in the terminally ill inherently makes the practice both distinct, and unmistakably imbued with sobriety.

The next best alternatives offered by the literature (sedation for intractable distress in the dying[13] or sedation in the imminently dying[14]) are more precise, but neither is likely to become part of medical jargon. Unabbreviated, they are cumbersome, and their acronyms (SIDD or SID), although easy enough to say,. are too similar to that of sudden infant death syndrome to avoid confusion. This leaves us with "palliative sedation," which is, of course, linguistically precise and clinically accurate. The etymology of the phrase implies sheltering (literally, "cloaking")[15] a patient from distress, via inducing a state of restfulness.

Surely, one might say, all this fuss over semantics is much ado about nothing. Hardly. Buber said that "what is within strives over and over again toward becoming language."[16] I have previously argued that the words we use in medical discourse reveal much about our truest conceptions (and subconscious assumptions) about the practice of the profession,[17] and have offered a set of internally consistent definitions of clinical terms often confused within the field of palliative medicine.[18] I suspect that in this case, as well, the linguistic ambiguity (and lack of clarity) of the phrase "terminal sedation" discloses similar moral ambiguity (and lack of clarity) surrounding the clinical practice. Let us take, therefore, this opportunity to clearly and firmly state that the goal of palliative sedation is the relief of suffering via the titration of medications to the cessation of symptoms-not the cessation of life. Socrates warned that using words carelessly was the kind of sin that kills the soul. Perhaps he was right,, for clarity of language can only follow, not precede, clarity of purpose and thought.

NOTES

1. P. Rousseau, "Existential suffering and palliative sedation: A brief commentary with a proposal for clinical guidelines," *Amer J Hosp & Palliat Care* 18, no. 3 (2001): 226–28; P. Rousseau, "Palliative sedation: A brief

review of ethical validity and clinical experience," *Mayo Clinic Proc* 75 (2000): 1064–69.

2. A. R. Jonsen, M. Siegler, and W. J. Winslade, *Clinical Ethics*, 4th ed. (New York: McGraw-Hill, 1998), pp. 1–208, passim.

3. R. E. Enck, "Drug-induced terminal sedation for symptom control," *Amer J Hosp & Palliat Care* 8, no. 5 (1991): 3–5.

4. B. M. Mount and P. Hamilton, "When palliative care fails to control suffering," *J Palliat Care* 10 (1994): 24–26.

5. J. A. Billings and S. D. Block, "Slow euthanasia," *J Palliat Care* 12 (1996): 21–30; A. A. Baker, "Slow euthanasia—or 'she will be better off in a hospital,'" *British Medical J* 2 (1976): 571–72.

6. J. Hallenbeck, "Terminal sedation: Ethical implications in different situations," *J Palliat Med* 3 (2000): 313–20; J. Hallenbeck, "Terminal sedation for intractable distress: Not slow euthanasia but a prompt response to suffering," *West J Med* 171 (1999): 222–23.

7. T. E. Quill, B. Lo, and D. W. Brock, "Palliative options of last resort: A comparison of voluntarily stopping eating and drinking, terminal sedation, physician-assisted suicide, and voluntary active euthanasia," *JAMA* 278 (1997): 2099–2104.

8. S. Chater et al., "Sedation for intractable distress in the dying: A survey of experts," *Palliat Med* 12 (1998): 255–69.

9. M. L. Yanow, Letter to the editor, *Ann Int Med* 133 (2000): 560; E. L. Krakauer, Letter to the editor, *Ann Int Med* 133 (2000): 560.

10. Hallenbeck, "Terminal sedation: Ethical implications in different situations," pp. 313–20; Hallenbeck, "Terminal sedation for intractable distress: Not slow euthanasia but a prompt response to suffering," pp. 222–23; T. E. Quill and I. R. Byock, "Responding to intractable terminal suffering: The role of terminal sedation and voluntary refusal of food and fluids," *Ann Int Med* 132 (2000): 408–14; J. Collins, "Case presentation: Terminal sedation in a pediatric patient," *J Pain Symp Mgmnt* 15 (1998): 258; J. L. Lynn, "Terminal sedation" Letter to the editor, *N Engl J Med* 338 (1998): 1230; D. Marquis, "The weakness of the case for legalizing physician-assisted suicide," in *Physician Assisted Suicide—Expanding the Debate*, ed. M. P. Battin, R. Rhodes, and A. Ailvers (New York: Routledge, 1998), pp. 267–78; E. J. Rosen, "A case of 'terminal sedation' in the family," *J Pain Symp Mgmt* 16 (1998): 406–407; Quill, Lo, and Brock, "Palliative options of last resort," pp. 2099–2104; M. Balfour, "Morphine drips, terminal seda-

tion, and slow euthanasia: Definitions and facts, not anecdotes," *J Palliat Care* 12 (1996): 31–37.

11. P. C. Rousseau, "Dying and terminal sedation," *Clin Geriatr* 7 (1999): 19–20.

12. Quill and Byock, Letter to the editor, *Ann Int Med* 133 (2000): 261–62.

13. Chater et al., "Sedation for intractable distress in the dying," pp. 255–69.

14. D. P. Sulmasy et al., Letter to the editor, *Ann Int Med* 133 (2000): 260–61.

15. *The Barnhart Concise Etymological Dictionary* (New York: Harper-Collins, 1995).

16. M. Buber, *The Knowledge of Man* (New York: Harper, 1965), p. 135.

17. W. C. Jackson, "In a word," *JAMA* 280 (1998): 493–94; W. C. Jackson, "Our best path forward," *Bioethics Forum* 14, no. 3/4 (1998): 49–51.

18. W. C. Jackson, "When all else is done: The challenge of improving antemortem care," Primary Care Companion to *J Clin Psych* 1 (1999): 146–53.

Part Three

SPIRITUAL CARE
FOR THE
DYING

1 3

SPIRITUALITY AND CARE
AT THE END OF LIFE

Myles N. Sheehan

W hat does it mean to attend to the spiritual needs of patients as they face serious illness? And what, if any, impact does a person's spirituality have on choices at the end of life? Does the openness of caregivers to a patient's spiritual experience affect their interaction with patients? Could explicit attention to spirituality help doctors and patients be frank about the goals of treatment and a person's choices about therapy?

DEFINITION OF SPIRITUALITY

Spirituality may conjure up a variety of images, some not at all flattering, and further definition is required. Philosophers, cognitive psychologists, and theologians have speculated endlessly about what it means to be human and about the nature and the

Reprinted from *Choices: The Newsletter of Choice in Dying* 6, no. 2 (summer 1997), by permission of Partnership for Caring, 1620 Eye Street, NW, Suite 202, Washington, D.C. 20006 (800) 989–9455.

interaction of body, mind, and spirit. Despite the complexity of the arguments, we humans are both body and spirit; we face life in ways that are more than physical reactions; and our understanding of what it means to be human includes a dimension that both encompasses and goes beyond our physicality.

There are at least three components to this spiritual dimension. First, spirituality is an expression of how a person relates to a larger whole, be it God, a higher power, the human family. Second, personal spirituality provides a source of meaning and understanding about the significance of being human. Third, personal spirituality often contains habits, rituals, gestures, and symbols that provide ways in which the person can interpret and manage existence.

Some physicians and others become quite nervous during any discussion of spirituality in medicine. They might fear that spirituality means enforcing particular religious beliefs. However, spirituality and religion are not synonymous. Religious belief is one very important way in which many people express their spirituality. But a person can be spiritual without explicit religious belief. Individuals have a variety of ways to find meaning in life; people come to an understanding of their choices and behaviors. And it is not uncommon to discover that a poem, a piece of music, or a good meal in the company of friends can provide a context by which one can grow, endure, or, even accept diminishment. Personal spirituality frequently is expressed by forms of religious practice. Faith provides a variety of personal and communal resources to handle serious illness. Serious illness causes believers and nonbelievers alike to face loss, fears, grief, personal mortality, and questions of meaning. These are the kind of issues that appropriately are identified, at least partially, as spiritual.

PHYSICIANS AND SPIRITUALITY

Why should doctors bother with spirituality? Three reasons are readily apparent. First, a doctor who inquires about a patient's spirituality gains a deeper insight into the patient's experience. Being a good doctor can be a bit like being a good reader. Doctors see, touch, hear, and participate in some of the most visceral parts of being human: birth, death, illness, recovery. They confront and can share in their patients' emotions of hope, despair, joy, and profound sorrow. Physicians look through the chapters of a person's life to gain access to a story that contains the mundane and the extraordinary. Doctors who miss the experience of the human spirit are like readers who skip several chapters in a book: they do not truly comprehend the whole because they have avoided crucial information.

Second, knowing all the chapters of a patient's story and thus gaining insight into that person's spiritual journey can provide a context for making medical decisions. As a person faces the end of life, the context can be especially crucial. For all the discussion and interest in informed consent, advance directives, and patients' rights, attempts to care for individuals at the end of life are often filled with poor communication and the inappropriate use of technology. This might well reflect the inability of doctors and patients to speak the same language. Doctors ask about ventilators, CPR, intubations, and feeding tubes. Patients and their families talk about death with dignity, refusing to give up, hopes for miracles, and requests to be left alone. If a physician understands a person's spiritual response to illness, better communication might result. Two examples may help illustrate the point. A person frightened about death, concerned about what will happen to a spouse and children, and despairing at the loss of hopes and dreams may cling to illusory hope about technology, or focus on the possible life-prolonging aspect of a particular therapy. The result could be an extensive period of aggressive care, the end result of which is increased suffering and death. A doctor who can ask about fears, hopes, and despair might be able to find the tools to ease the spiritual pain without blindly resorting to invasive treatments that will not bring the patient the peace he or she seeks. Likewise, an individual who has come to the end of an illness can communicate to a physician spiritual acceptance of mortality. The doctor is in a better position to discuss care that is compatible with the person's view of the dying process.

A third reason doctors should be concerned about a patient's spiritual experience is that it allows doctors to help patients in a way that is fundamental to medicine: limiting suffering and not abandoning patients to the experience of illness. As people die, they could be in spiritual distress as deep as any physical pain. Allowing the patient to express spiritual pain is one way to help heal a person's spirit, especially when physical cure is impossible. Helping a patient find spiritual resources and assistance is another way of providing care. Arranging a meeting with a chaplain, facilitating a call to a clergy person, or allowing the patient and family to pray and conduct devotions in a hospital environment can succor a patient who is in pain and at the end of life. Likewise, an awareness of and respect for common religious practices around death and dying are integral parts of compassionate care for terminally ill patients. Ritual and prayer are important vehicles by which the human spirit finds meaning in and transcends grief, pain, and loss. For example, a doctor who does not know how to show respect for the body of an Orthodox Jew at the time of death or who is ignorant about the meaning and power of the Sacrament of the Sick for Roman Catholics lacks key ways to diminish the spiritual suffering of patients and families.

How do doctors and other caregivers access the spirituality of their patients? Three simple suggestions provide a starting point. One, do not avoid the subject if patients discuss questions of meaning or their need for specific religious practices. Two, ask simple questions: Can you help me to understand what it has been like for you to be sick? What have you found hardest to cope with? What are your sources of strength? What keeps you going? Is God or religion important to you as you face your illness? Three, willingly help patients and families find spiritual resources if they so desire.

OBSTACLES

Obstacles and problems occur in integrating spirituality with medicine. Physicians might be reluctant to get involved with questions that make them uncomfortable and that they have failed to address personally, although it is unlikely that a doctor who has not confronted the possibility of personal illness and death would be good at caring for very ill people. Second, a profound ignorance about spiritually and religion exists in America. Because of this ignorance, some will seek to find a conflict between the scientific practice of medicine and topics like spirituality and religion. Neither belief in the human spirit nor faith in God implies antipathy toward science or an advocacy of nontraditional medicine. Third, some sensationalize the topic of spirituality in medicine, suggesting a lunatic fringe appeal. The media often focus on spectacular claims of faith healing, alleged miracles, and extraordinary experiences, rather than on a doctor's simple concern about his or her patient's response to illness, fears, hopes, and source of meaning in life and death. Obstacles and problems aside, however, recognizing the spiritual side to illness opens up new dimensions for caring.

REDISCOVERY

Is there really anything particularly new about spirituality in medicine? Probably not. It is more a rediscovery of something that was once taken for granted. Before doctors had much in the way of technology, they knew how to attend their patients even when little could be done in the face of disease or serious illness. Now that doctors have a variety of ways to care for people, including life-saving and life-prolonging high-technology treatments, we must rediscover ways to care for the human spirit.

14

SPIRITUAL CARE
AT THE END OF LIFE

Tad Dunne

Those who care for the nonmedical needs of the dying must attend to their patients on at least four different levels at once—emotional, ethical, religious, and spiritual. For years, the spiritual level had been considered part of the other three. Many caregivers simply identified the spiritual with the religious or tacitly assumed that the ethical or emotional issues covered the other-than-bodily concerns of the dying.

But recently we find religious people protesting that their spiritual needs are not met by their religion, nor by anything in ethics or psychology, and nonreligious people raising questions about issues they call "spiritual." Not long ago in these pages, in fact, John Hardwig challenged bioethicists to look more closely at spiritual care.[1] At life's end, he observed, the dying usually return to long-neglected questions about what really counts in life. Many see little meaning in their narrowed and shortened future as they are forced to deal with friends and family in new and embarrassing ways. Where formerly they helped to lift burdens from the shoulders of

Reprinted from *The Hastings Center Report* 31, no. 2 (March/April 2001): 22–26.

others, they have now become a burden. They feel betrayed by their own bodies. They picture themselves as cast out from the society of the healthy. They can be overwhelmed by their feelings of isolation and abandonment, even self-hatred, fear, and anger.

True, most caregivers recognize these needs as "spiritual," but few know how to respond to them effectively, whether they are the family members of a dying parent or professional pastoral care workers. Caregivers need words and ideas to guide the attention they pay. Field instructors in training programs need to clarify how the spiritual needs of the dying relate to their emotional, ethical, and religious needs. Hospice administrators need criteria for hiring effective caregivers. For all these domains of care, we need a more precise articulation of the spiritual.

WHAT IS "THE SPIRITUAL"?

To move the discussion a step toward that precision, I suggest we think of the spiritual as involving the ways we transcend ourselves that are not based on reason alone. Or to chisel more precision out of that amorphous term *reason*, we can think of the spiritual as that realm of our living that goes beyond the insights and values that we can easily explain. I don't mean to suggest that reason has no place in spirituality. We strategize, we plan, we analyze, we weigh pros and cons, we test our ideas on experience, we use logic to make sure we're being consistent and clear. But people facing death are concerned less with what they can account for and more with their hopes, their companionships, and all the happy, baffling decisions they made that opened up to them a richer and deeper life.

It seems to me that this is what we mean when we refer to "the spiritual." We are speaking of "ultimate meaning." We are speaking of all the ways we are drawn toward a "beyond" throughout our lives, despite the fact that we never fully understand it. I'm thinking of transcendent events: How art and music symbolize the harmonies that we seek. How falling in love means taking risks that a rational assessment would not warrant. How I might realize that the expression "There's more to this than meets the eye" is actually true about everything. How the questions about God and eternity occur even to militant atheists. Poetry can convey it:

> Like pond-bound fish under global vaults of air,
> Speckled by beams from up beyond our sight,
> Whence luster menaces yet entices,
> What shall we make of the light?

Several sages, widely separated in history, identified three remarkably similar ways we approach these transcendent meanings. Heraclitus considered faith, hope, and charity as modes of knowledge distinct from a *cognitio rationis*.[2] St. Paul pointed to these three modes as bringing him to true wisdom in Christ Jesus. Although Paul is the only biblical author who mentions this triad, the fact that it has become enshrined as the theological virtues familiar to Christians today suggests that they represent recognizably distinct features of our consciousness. Bernard Lonergan, without appealing to any religious doctrines, demonstrated that any real solution to human evil had to be a kind of faith, a kind of hope, and a kind of charity.[3] Lonergan went further than Heraclitus and Paul by giving a functional explanation of exactly how these events make us self-transcending. That is, he was not laying out faith, hope, and charity as just cognitive elements in some epistemology. Nor was he proposing them as standards for religious living. Rather he was explaining how they already operate in everyone's consciousness to deal with ultimate meanings. His empirical approach seems to me to meet a criterion J. Hardwig sets out for any definition of the spiritual, namely, that it should make sense to nonreligious people yet not exclude religious meanings.

Faith, Lonergan says, is the knowledge born of transcendent love.[4] By transcendent love, Lonergan means yielding to the pull toward beauty, intelligibility, truth, value, and company without restriction. He underscores that these transcendentals have no intrinsic limitations—we can always seek more—and whether or not we conceptualize our yielding in religious terms, when we so yield, there is no end to the values we are open to recognizing. This yielding love becomes explicitly religious when we recognize ultimate values in a Torah, a Christ, a Koran, or a Buddha and decide to follow their lead in a community of like-minded believers.

For evidence that transcendent love is an independent source of knowledge, Lonergan cites Blaise Pascal's celebrated observation that the heart has reasons unknown to reason. The knowledge here is primarily a knowledge of values, and only as a result is it a set of truths. When we share love, we reprioritize what we appreciate and what we disparage in the world around us. We see eternal worth in another person; we more quickly recognize a value-rich community when we see one; we more keenly discern which of our heart's many inspirations we should follow. We feel empowered to be civil to the uncivil. We take on responsibilities that logic tells us to avoid. Our knowledge of values results in a set of truths—the knowledge of facts we take on belief rather than proof, because we trust the word of those we love. By liberating our minds and hearts to see higher meanings, deeper values, and saving truths, faith lies at the heart of any social or political policies aimed at bringing out the best in us.

Such a functional view of faith seems a better approach to talking about spirituality. It avoids identifying faith with religious truths, yet it underlies what every religious person holds true. It also avoids a strict identification of faith with trust in God, yet it includes a trust in transcendent reality by whatever name one knows it.

Along the same lines, hope can be defined as desire rendered confident by this faith.[5] Hope is a desire, not a certitude; a yearning, not a possession. It is confident because transcendent love moves us to believe, often in the face of horrendously contrary evidence, that the world is not ultimately senseless and that morality is far more than obedience or convention.

Having hope is not the same as having hopes. While we achieve some of our hopes and fall short of others, none of them has the ultimacy that makes further hope either superfluous or futile. Those who are dying, in particular, can glow with hope even when their lives are littered with disappointments. Hope is a transcendent kind of knowledge because it anticipates a beyond, a resolution of all chaos, and an ultimate meaning to the universe whatever our personal role in it.

Because our minds cannot formulate what this beyond is like, we rely on our imagination to represent it to ourselves. We imagine what our family could be. We visualize world peace. We surround ourselves with symbols of transcendence: the image of blindfolded Justice with her scales; the statue we call Liberty; and the architectural renderings of facades that suggest Security in a bank and Wisdom in a university.

Religious hope works the same way in our consciousness, but it has an explicit object. We imagine God and our life with God. We create sacraments as palpable media for connecting with a God who is Spirit. We paint or carve the images that focus our attention on the divine. We compose the music that lifts our hearts to the ultimately transcendent. We write rubrics for reenacting and celebrating holy moments. We design churches whose lines and spaces point to the obscure object of our yearning.

Such confident desire can enable a society to withstand the pressures of greed and revenge that precipitate wars. It can energize the individual to try; and try again, in the face of broken friendships, bankruptcy, or the string of slow losses that come with age. It gives healing time for the vision of faith to reverse enmities and gradually build the social systems that reflect human dignity. This functional view of hope can make sense to anyone, religious or not.

The third mode of spiritual transcendence is charity. In Lonergan's analysis, only a species of charity will halt the spiral of retribution that prolongs wars, breaks families, and drags civility down to barbarism. Charity releases us from the prisons of our unchallenged opinions by exposing us to the viewpoints of others. It raises questions in us that we never thought of, and it opens up new worlds to us when we find some answers. It is the spirit of charity that makes a couple out of two egos, a family out of a couple, a neighborhood out of families, a people out of neighborhoods. Charity is no picnic, of course, since we always lose some ego when we embrace the compromises that mutual love entails. Hesitate we may, but we are also drawn. This charity, then, is not first a standard that ethics upholds; it is first an impulse, an allure, and an invitation. We recognize this pull as ultimate because we know very well it could take us anywhere.

The acts of charity are the same for both the religious and nonreligious. Even the felt motivation is practically the same. A religious woman does not love her neighbor for a religious reason; she feels an impulse to love and she obeys. While she believes that this love is God's gift, she also recognizes that it is ultimately love that makes her life and death meaningful.

SPIRITUAL ISSUES OF DYING

These three major ways we connect to ultimate meanings suggest some preliminary conclusions about spiritual care at the end of life. But first a caution. Over the centuries, the terms *faith, hope,* and *charity* have become exclusively religious. To keep our focus wide enough to include nonreligious perspectives, I suggest we translate these virtues into three correlative "issues." For faith, the issue is commitments; for hope, aesthetics, and for charity, company.

First, consider how commitments are an expression of faith. Faith—the values we embrace out of transcendent love—shows in our commitments. It does not show in every commitment, but only in those in which our decisions are motivated chiefly by love. We all have memories of taking a risk because we trusted someone's word out of love. Whether this love was for God, for a friend, or even for a community to whom we felt loyal, in many of the major turns in our lives, we pivoted on our hearts, not our minds. We may recall decisions to protest injustice or to defend the status quo, to marry and raise a family or to live in celibate community, to switch careers or to stay the course. In conversations with people facing death, these are important events—how big a risk they took, how trusting they were, how courageously they met life's challenges. These form the golden threads gleaming in every person's biography, tying together the lists of places they lived, the awards they received, the people they met.

These stories beg telling as death approaches. Many people have no experience talking about their commitments. They just made them, carried by a deep-running love that seemed like still waters to bystanders. Pastoral caregivers need to raise the topic and learn how to pursue it, more delicately with those who show no interest in spiritual things, but persistently. Other people facing death feel an acute sense of having *avoided* commitments that their hearts recommended. This too is about ultimate meaning in their lives, and caregivers can help them address it. The mere willingness to listen can heal this moral wound much like fresh air heals a skin abrasion.

Imagine a woman who admits having avoided religious commitment. That doesn't mean she never let herself be moved by love, nor that she consciously foreclosed all thought of ultimates. At a minimum, effective care can focus on how she followed her heart, particularly on what her heart valued above all, whether or not she names it God.

It is important to keep in mind that the work of giving spiritual care occurs originally and essentially within the caregivers. They need to keep a few central questions in mind about the person before them—questions posed mainly to themselves. Regarding faith, the caregiver's central question about the dying person might be, In what circumstances did she let her heart take the lead?

Next, consider how aesthetic experience is related to hope. Usually, it takes images to enkindle hope, to represent those things we long for. Ideas, concepts, and logic leave the heart cold. Images, however, are not the only vehicle of hope. Any raw experience that represents hoped-for possibilities will work, as long as these experiences are palpable, significant to the individual, and aesthetically inviting. For the eye, we need windows that open out on luminous landscapes, artwork with magnetic staying power, rooms and furniture pleasing to the eye and rich in reminders of the transcendent riches of home or healing or adventure or safety. For the ear, we need places of silence, places where nature can be heard, and listening places for music that lifts the spirit. For the hand, we need to notice the textures and the weight of things, considering what deep associations might arise when the dying person handles them. For the foot, we need to understand what walking means for people who cannot walk far: for them too it is of profound symbolic importance to stand at a threshold, to venture out, to turn a corner, to explore, or to make it to the sink. Whether a man sways in a little dance or abbreviates a genuflection, he exercises hope. For the nose, we need places where the smell of urine and feces are contained behind a dignifying bathroom door and evacuated by a good fan. For the tongue, the image of eating is literally a matter of taste. Tomato soup usually says "home" to an American, but not to the Japanese. For a man in Milwaukee, drinking means beer; for a woman in Toronto, wine. For some, eating means company; for others it's just nourishment.

Obviously, environment counts, whether for nursing homes or hospice facilities or the dying person's home. It requires sensitive attention to individual tastes. Some will want Mozart, others silence. Some want a view of nature, others art classics. Sometimes, an individual's apparent tastes mask deeper needs. When, say, a dying man's tastes lean to mindless television, a caregiver's gift is to probe deeper to uncover more effective symbols of hope. The caregiver's central question might be: What images and experiences give this person hope?

Finally, consider that the essence of charity is found in human company. Charity has unfortunately come to mean just giving to others, something we do easily for fame or a tax deduction. But real charity is both to give *and* to receive. It means entering a relationship without control of its future, and not all relationships embody this unnerving sacrifice of control. Many relationships with colleagues or siblings have little transcendence about them. What distinguishes charity is how it weaves a network of *companions in the struggle*—a company of those who share a sense of the mystery of life, of a common concern for progeny, and of a final destiny that awaits them together.

The love they feel does not have to be restricted to the living. The elderly in particular feel company with friends who have died. Nor should this love be restricted to humans. Religious people need to talk about their love for God and God's love for them. And even nonreligious people can swell with gratitude for the gift of being able to love without necessarily thanking God.

Caregivers need to be on the lookout for those who really are the main characters in the dying person's transcendent drama, since personas often get in the way. More than eliciting stories, though, caregivers also need to be aware of the paradoxical birth of a new charity just as physical death draws closer—the palpable company that the dying person and the caregiver share in this struggle. Their mutual presence is charity alive; it is a common presence to mystery; and though it doesn't need to be talked about, it is important for both parties to feel the blessing and the gift. Aware of the present moment, then, and of the dying person's companions in life's mystery, the caregiver's central question might be, Whose company made her a better person?

PLANNING ACCORDINGLY

The essential work of providing spiritual care falls first on the caregivers. To notice the spiritual needs of the dying, they need to be familiar with these transcendent events. Some may object that they can get this only secondhand, by attending to what dying people express. But all self-transcendence involves dying because life's decisions always involve a dying to alternatives. Indeed, in our major life decisions we frequently experience the adjustments that Elisabeth Kübler-Ross spelled out about the dying—denial, depression, bargaining, anger, and acceptance. In these decisions, anyone who cannot see values beyond their logic, mystery beyond their lives, and people beyond their egos will by default act on mere consistency or pure compulsion. The more they recognize the death in every moment, the better company they will be to the dying and the more readily will they learn life lessons from them. Fortunately, we now and then meet a magnificent tutor—the dying person whose attitude teaches us about living with deep awareness of ultimate meanings.

A practical service that a caregiver can give is to help those who are dying tell their stories. This requires an ability to drill down beneath the work histories and the photo albums to uncover the transcendent decisions that committed them to some liberating path in life and to name those friends with whom they shared a keen awareness of a beyond. Even with religious people, it is important to peel back their religious practices and uncover their commitments and company, including and especially the company they keep with God. The primary payoff here is to help the dying become more aware and more appreciative of the spiritual dimensions of their lives. However, there's a valuable secondary payoff as well. By recording these stories—by audio or videotape or by writing a biography based on interview notes—surviving family and friends inherit a poignant record of the spiritual depths of their loved one.

Transcendent concerns cannot be met without the practical work of raising money to support this kind of care. It costs money to hire specialists in pastoral care and to create the aesthetic environments of hospice or home that keep hope alive. Fund-raisers and advertising help, but given the influence of the old saw, "If you can't quantify it, it doesn't exist," we also need to support empirical studies that will allow the transcendent needs of the dying to be reasonably compared to their medical and emotional needs. In the long run, probably, funds will be available only to the extent that specific communities of people, whose loved ones include those with terminal cancer, leukemia, AIDS, end-stage renal disease, multiple sclerosis, or the like, become aware of these spiritual needs and join the discussion of how to allocate available healthcare funds. Education on the ancient triad of commitment, aesthetics, and company will keep the question of spiritual needs alive and build a foundation for further insights and growing awareness among the general public.

NOTES

1. J. Hardwig, "Spiritual issues at the end of life: A call for discussion," *Hastings Center Report* 30, no. 2 (2000): 28–30; see also C. B. Cohen et al., "Prayer as therapy," *Hastings Center Report* 30, no. 3 (2000): 40–47.

2. The philosopher Eric Voegelin noted this feature of Heraclitus's thought. See E. Webb, *Eric Voegelin: Philosopher of History* (Seattle: University of Washington Press, 1981), p. 115. Voegelin points out that these different dimensions of knowing are not readily distinguished in ordinary experience.

3. B. Lonergan, *Method in Theology* (New York. Herder & Herder, 1972), pp. 117–18. The triad of a saving faith, hope, and charity occurs in a number of Lonergan's works. A more thorough presentation of the functional significance of faith, hope, and charity can be found in *Insight: A Study of Human Understanding*, vol. 3 of *Collected Works of Bernard Lonergan* (Toronto: University of Toronto Press, 1992), pp. 718–51.

4. See Lonergan, *Method in Theology*, p. 115. Lonergan's actual definition runs, "Faith is the knowledge born of religious love." The careful reader will note that by religious, Lonergan does not identify this love with what a person feels who claims to be religious. Underneath what we call religious expression, religious love is a prior apprehension of tran-

scendent value. "This apprehension consists in the experienced fulfill-ment of our unrestricted thrust to self-transcendence, in our actuated orientation toward the mystery of love and awe." I have substituted the term *transcendent* for *religious* to keep in our scope those people who may be deeply committed to transcendent love and yet do not consider themselves "religious."

5. See T. Dunne, *Lonergan and Spirituality* (Chicago: Loyola University Press, 1985), pp. 123–26.

15

CONTROL THEORY
IN DYING
What Do We Know?

Susan Redding

CONTROL AT THE END OF LIFE

Numerous studies attest to the fact that America is in a state of crisis over the way we provide care for those among us who are dying.[1] A common theme among these studies is the apparent lack of control held at the end of life by patients or their appointed surrogates. Both the professional and lay communities have responded to this crisis in care for the dying with several initiatives. Passage of the Patient Self-Determination Act in 1991 gave Americans legal rights to guide interventions at the end of their lives. Programs such as Last Acts, The Project on Death in America, Supportive Care of the Dying, and the Missoula Demonstration Project are examining how we might improve our care for the dying. As we struggle, as a society, to find a better way to provide care at the end of life, it is imperative that we remember that death belongs to the dying. The only person who can inform us, on an

Reprinted from *American Journal of Hospice & Palliative Care* 17, no. 3 (May/June 2000): 204–208.

existential level, of what is needed at the end of life is the individual who is dying.

This article will explore the issue of control for the dying. A brief historical perspective and review of control theory as it relates to health will be followed by a review of the literature related to patients' perceptions of the role of control at the end of life.

HISTORICAL PERSPECTIVES

Since the Middle Ages, control by dying persons over their lives until death has gradually diminished.[2] Several social trends have contributed to this phenomenon. The "prolongevity revolution," spurred by the development of technological medicine, and the institutionalization of the dying have altered the face of death. In the late eighteenth century, doctors began to replace priests at the bedside, implying that death was a physical rather than a spiritual process and dealt with more effectively by medicine than by prayer.[3] Eighty to 90 percent of people at that time, and until the early 1900s, died in their homes. As death moved into institutions, families lost touch with both the dying and how to care for them; the dying, once they were institutionalized, were severely limited from controlling their own lives. Moreover, the dying found themselves isolated by death-denying professionals who viewed dying as stark evidence of their powerlessness and their failure to utilize science to stop the death trajectory. "Social death preceded physiological extinction.[4]

Additional medical and social phenomena have contributed to the current crisis in care of the dying. The increasing reliance on specialists for medical care, the growing absence of traditional caregivers, federal regulations and policies, and the demand for efficiency and profitability in healthcare have all played their part. Indeed, the current battle with death continues to focus on the body and on discovering technical solutions to the problem of death despite mounting evidence that we cannot continue to place unlimited faith in technology as the solution to human problems.[5] "For the dying individual, the medicalization of death has resulted in de-individualization and loss of control."[6]

CONTROL THEORY

Belief in control over one's life may be the most important defense against the experience of distress for the individual.[7] R. Schultz and B. H. Hanusa see perceived choice and a sense of personal control as the critical determinants of older adults' physical and psychological well-being.[8] J. Mirowsky and C. Ross[9] identify powerlessness as the expectation of the individual that her or his behavior cannot determine the outcomes sought; in other words, it is the belief that the individual has no control over outcomes. Powerlessness can be demoralizing in itself and often decreases the motivation to cope effectively with difficult life situations.

Control theory holds that active, effective problem solving contributes to the development of a sense of well-being. Additionally, those with a sense of internal control experience less depression.[10] Undesirable events in which the individual has played some part and shared some responsibility are less distressing than uncontrollable negative events. Mere belief in control, even if not exerted, lessens the negative consequences of exposure to uncontrollable events.[11] Arthur Kleinman reminds us of the cross-cultural presence of the need for control. In societies as diverse as Puritan New England and tribal Africa, witchcraft became the explanatory model for malignant illnesses that were random and unpredictable. Witchcraft offered a magical means to exert some control over seemingly unjust suffering and untimely death.[12] In summary, the conditions that rob people of control in their lives increase distress.[13]

THE SENSE OF CONTROL AND ILLNESS

How we respond psychologically and behaviorally to a physical illness can affect the intensity and duration of the symptoms of that illness.[14] When that physical illness is terminal, the individual also faces one of the most stressful developmental events in life.[15] How can what we know about control theory help us to assist people approaching the end of life, when continued control over one's life becomes increasingly difficult?

We know human beings exposed to stress cope better if they feel they have control.[16] People who have a sense of personal control exhibit better physical health overall. In N. Krause and S. Stryker's review of literature on locus of control, stress, and well-being, the common referent was the subjective feeling of the individual that she or he could effectively direct his/her own life.[17] Rose Weitz's study of AIDS patients supports the hypothesis that the key to coping with the uncertainty of that disease is having a sense of control.[18]

Lack of control translates into a sense of powerlessness. Norman Cousins purports that the sense of powerlessness is so strong a negative force that it should be considered a disease in itself.[19] Body mechanisms involved with a sense of lack of control cause stress and depression and may actually wear and destroy body tissue.[20] The effect of the psyche on the soma is supported by research in the field of psychoimmunology. Individuals exhibiting what Aaron Antonovsky identified as a sense of coherence can activate immune cells to fight cancer.[21] This sense of coherence includes a feeling of confidence that the environment is structured and predictable, that resources are available to cope with the demands imposed by it, and that dealing with these demands is worth the effort. The sense of coherence enables one to have some control in dealing with one's environment. The sense of control has powerful implications for wellness and healing in human beings.

WHAT DO THE DYING SAY ABOUT CONTROL?

Dorothy Caruso-Herman identifies loss of control as perhaps the major concern of dying persons.[22] Donna Burgess further reinforces the importance of control for the terminally ill when she notes that loss of control in illness can be overwhelming and may encompass loss of personal identity, relationships, physical abilities, sexual capabilities, self-care ability, and potential future. The normal reaction to loss of control is an effort to regain some control.[23] Research findings confirm that maintenance of control is an important issue for dying persons and their loved ones. Peter Singer et al., in a qualitative study involving 126 seriously ill patients, attempted to identify elements of quality-of-life care from the perspective of these patients. Not only was achieving a sense of control identified as one of five domains of quality end-of-life care, but patients were adamant that they or their proxy retain this control until death.[24] These findings were supported by Merrijoy Kelner's research with both healthy and seriously ill elderly persons. Of the well elderly, 90 percent stated they wanted control at the time of their deaths. Of the thirty-eight seriously ill patients Kelner interviewed, 71 percent expressed the desire to exercise control over medical decisions made at the end of their lives. Although most of these patients wanted control to avoid clinical decisions that would prolong their lives beyond their wishes, a few (four) wanted to ensure that everything would be done to keep them alive. Only 1 percent of this sample would find physician-assisted suicide acceptable for themselves. Those patients who did not express a desire for control at the end of life, were reluctant to talk of dying and felt it inappropriate to consider who should make end-of-life decisions. Demographically, those elderly most likely to desire control of end-of-life decision making were better educated and more likely to be in middle or higher social classes. The author projects that future generations are more likely to fall in this cohort.[25]

Interviews with forty-eight patients undergoing hemodialysis who had completed an advanced directive indicated they had done so to exercise control of their dying and to relieve burdens on loved ones. In the words of one participant, "It's all written down there, what I want. It makes me feel secure."[26] Oncology nurses relate descriptions of patients' attempts to exert some degree of control at the end of life. These nurses report that a patient's fear is not of death but of loss of independence, dignity, and the sense of control that gives meaning to the quality of life.[27] As an explanation for what had been labeled as her "inappropriate behavior," one patient stated, "When you feel like you're losing control over everything . . . you get kind of crazy."[28]

Despite compelling evidence from the literature on the influence of a sense of control on well-being, and the fact that control is described as one of six criteria for an appropriate death,[29] documented studies indicate that control is not within the grasp of most dying persons. Research findings suggest that the vast outlays of resources for life-extending technologies at the end of life are not driven by patient demand.[30] This phenomenon raises the issue of who has the right or obligation to use technology to prolong death or sustain life and under what circumstances.[31] Ira Byock supports the notion that dying is a fundamentally personal experience, not a set of medical problems to be solved.[32] Readers of a professional gerontological nursing journal were asked to identify experiences contributing to "a good death" or a positive process of dying. Respondents asserted that the process of dying was positive if the individuals involved perceived it to be so, supporting the concept of "a good death" as a subjective and personal experience.[33] Who better to control a fundamentally personal experience than the person involved? Thompson maintains that we should use the benefits of science to provide the dying with a nurturing spiritual environment that feeds the spirit while sustaining the body.[34]

IMPLICATIONS FOR CARE

The patient's right to choose is well supported. Current ethical and legal opinions amply affirm that upon the request of a competent patient or patient surrogate, the physician is obligated to withhold or withdraw life-sustaining treatment, including respirators, chemotherapy, antibiotics, and/or blood transfusions. The American Society of Clinical Oncology's Task Force on Cancer Care at the End of Life has outlined several principles upon which to base a humane system of care. Responsiveness to patients' wishes is one of these four principles. The American Medical Association Institute for Ethics has identified eight elements of quality end-of-life care. Among these are the opportunity to discuss and plan end-of-life care, assurance that preferences for withholding or withdrawing life-sustaining interventions will be honored, and attention to the personal goals of the dying process.[35] Despite these guidelines and others like them, many persons express uncertainty about whether their wishes at the end of life will be honored. In fact, the statistics support this concern.

Patients report several possible barriers to maintenance of control regarding end-of-life decisions—including family members or caregivers, physicians, and religious leaders.[36] Despite the fact that patient control is central to the hospice concept of care, studies in these settings indicate that up to two-thirds of hospice professionals have difficulty relinquishing control.[37] Mesler states that the principle of increased patient control highlights the classic tensions between autonomy and paternalism in medicine.[38] The most important concern for patients and families may be for professional caregivers to validate their feelings and allow them to make choices.[39]

To respond more effectively to patient and family needs, healthcare professionals will need to assist them to gain a sense of control over distressing symptoms at the end of life. The presence of physical symptoms at this time is highly correlated with increased depression, distress, and anxiety.[40] Healthcare professionals will need to recognize that anger, withdrawal, and depression may be patient responses to loss of control. In a study of awareness of dying, Clive Seale et al. found that those dying in open awareness (dying person and family caregiver both know patient is dying) had more opportunity for emotional closeness and control over the circumstances of the death.[41] The positive effect of a good dying experience, where family caregivers feel the patient was given choices about treatment, cannot be overlooked.[42]

Specific environments can be enabling or constraining factors in fostering patient control at the end of life. For example, institutional or agency policies can control the duration and frequency of visits or the availability of resources for clients. Environments that are constraining can greatly limit the effectiveness of interventions aimed at the individual.[43] Those planning interventions to improve end-of-life care will need to be alert to the effects of the environment on the attainment of their goals.

In our efforts as practitioners to alleviate distress for the patient, it is important to acknowledge that, despite ideal treatment, the patient's suffering may persist. Suffering cannot always be eradicated and may not be an inappropiate experience as one approaches the end of one's life. The well-meaning attempts by others of totally eliminating suffering for the dying person may come with unintended consequences. Courtney Campbell attests that efforts by patients, their advocates, or professionals to efface suffering will come at a cost to mortal humanity. Individuals will risk losing those traits of identity and integrity that make them who they are: ". . . to relieve patients of fundamental features of the human condition can itself be dehumanizing."[44] Byock reminds us that an examination of the experience of dying would be incomplete without exploring the nature of opportunity at the end of life. "Some people emerge from the depths of suffering— and the virtual disintegration of the person they once were—to report a sense of wellness as they are dying."[45]

CONCLUSION

"Creative ideas and inventions are born from problems coupled with imagination."[46] How we utilize advances in the sciences to create more caring and nurturing possibilities for dying remains to be seen. The model we develop will be the product of multiple forces at work in our society. Perhaps the solution will come from the dying themselves. In the words of L. M. Thompson:

> In gaining a sense of control over our own medical treatments, in making conscious choices about how we spend our lives, and in allowing others into our suffering, we are releasing innate healing capacities that make us nature's allies in our own recovery.[47]

As we struggle, as a society, to develop a model for wellness in dying, one truth is certain—"the future of death is secure."[48]

NOTES

1. I. Byock, *Dying Well: The Prospect for Growth at the End of Life* (New York: Riverhead Books, 1997); SUPPORT Principal Investigators, "A controlled trial to improve care for seriously ill hospitalized patients," *JAMA* 274, no. 20 (1995): 1591–98; H. G. Prigerson, "Socialization to dying: Social determinants of death acknowledgment and treatment among terminally ill geriatric patients," *J Health & Soc Behav* 33 (1992): 378–95; S. L. Taylor, "Quandary at the crossroads: Paternalism versus advocacy surrounding end of life treatment decisions," *Amer J Hosp Palliat Care* 12, no. 4 (1995): 43–47; L. M. Thompson, "The future of death: Death in the hands of science," *Nursing Outlook* 42, no. 4 (1994): 175–80.

2. P. Aries, *The Hour of Our Death* (New York: Alfred A. Knopf, 1995).

3. T. Walter, "Natural death and the noble savage," *Omega* 30, no. 4 (1995): 237–48.

4. A. Rinaldi and M. C. Kearl, "The hospice farewell: Idiological perspectives of its professional practitioners," *Omega* 21, no. 4 (1990): 283–300.

5. Thompson, "The future of death," pp. 175–80.

6. Rinaldi and Kearl, "The hospice farewell," pp. 283–300.

7. J. Mirowsky and C. E. Ross, "Social patterns of distress," *Ann Rev Soc* 12 (1986): 23–45; A. Antonovsky, *Unraveling the Mystery of Health* (San Francisco: Jossey-Bass, 1987); R. Weitz, "Uncertainty and the lives of people with AIDS," in *Readings in Medical Sociology*, ed. W. C. Cockerman, M. Glasser, and L. S. Heuser (Upper Saddle River, N.J.: Prentice-Hall, 1998); P. A. Thoist, "Stress, coping, and social support processes: Where are we? What next?" in *Readings in Medical Sociology*, ed. W. C. Cockerman, Glasser, and Heuser.

8. R. Schultz and B. H. Hanusa, "Experimental social gerontology: A social psychological perspective," *J Soc Iss* 36, no. 2 (1980): 30–46.

9. Mirowsky and Ross, "Social patterns of distress," pp. 23–45.

10. J. Mirowsky and C. E. Ross, "Control or defense? Depression and the sense of control over good and bad outcomes," *J Health Soc Behav* 31 (1990): 71–86.

11. D. C. Glass and J. E. Singer, "Behavioral aftereffects of unpredictable and uncontrollable aversive events," *American Scientist* 60, no. 4 (1972): 457–65.

12. A. Kleinman, *The Illness Narratives: Suffering, Healing, and the Human Condition* (New York: Basic Books, 1988).

13. Mirowsky and Ross, "Social patterns of distress," pp. 23–45.

14. R. Schultz and J. Schlarb, "Two decades of research on dying: What do we know about the patient?" *Omega* 18, no. 4 (1987): 299–317.

15. L. Paton, "The sacred circle: A conceptual framework for spiritual care in hospice," *Amer J Hosp Palliat Care* 13 (1996): 52–56.

16. Antonovsky, *Unraveling the Mystery of Health*; Weitz, "Uncertainty and the lives of people with AIDS."

17. N. Cousins, *Anatomy of an Illness* (Boston: Hall, 1979).

18. Weitz, "Uncertainty and the lives of people with AIDS."

19. Cousins, *Anatomy of an Illness.*

20. Paton, "The sacred circle," pp. 52–56; C. Peterson and J. Seligman, "Causal explanations as a risk factor for depression: Theory and evidence," *Psych Rev* 91 (1984): 783–90; M. Seeman and T. E. Seeman, "Health behavior and personal autonomy: A longitudinal study of the sense of control in illness," *J Health Soc Behav* 24 (1983): 144–60.

21. Mirowsky and Ross, "Social patterns of distress," pp. 23–45; J.

Post-White, "The role of sense of coherence in mediating the effects of mental imagery on immune function, cancer outcomes, and quality of life," in *Sense of Coherence and Resiliency: Stress, Coping, and Health*, eds. H. I. McCubbin et al. (Madison: University of Wisconsin System, 1994).

22. D. Caruso-Herman, "Concerns for the dying patient and family," *Seminars Onc Nurs* 5, no. 2 (1989): 120–23.

23. D. Burgess, "Denial and terminal illness," *Amer J Hosp & Palliat Care* 11, no. 2 (1994): 46–48.

24. P. A. Singer, D. K. Martin, and M. Kelner, "Quality end of life care: Patients' perspectives," *JAMA* 281, no. 2 (1999): 163–68.

25. M. Kelner, "Activists and delegators: Elderly patients' preferences about control at the end of life," *Soc Science & Med* 41, no. 4 (1995): 537–45.

26. P. A. Singer et al., "Reconceptualizing advanced care planning from the patient's perspective," *Arch Int Med* 158 (1994): 879–84.

27. L. Matuk, "Choices," *Canadian Nurse* 87, no. 6 (1991): 30–31.

28. Y. Arnell, "An ounce of control," *Nursing92* 22, no. 4 (1992): 83.

29. A. Weisman, "Appropriate death and the hospice program," *Hospice Journal* 4, no. 1 (1988): 66–70.

30. Prigerson, "Socialization to dying," pp. 378–95.

31. M. Olsen, *Healing the Dying* (Albany, N.Y.: Delmar Publishing, 1997).

32. Byock, *Dying Well*.

33. C. Kovach, "In your practice, what experiences of patients and family members could be classified as 'a good death' or a positive process of dying?" *J Gerontol Nurs* 24, no. 7 (1998): 47–52.

34. Thompson, "The future of death," pp. 175–80.

35. ASCO, Task Force on Cancer Care at the End of Life, "Cancer care during the last phase of life," *J Clin Onc* 16, no. 5 (1998): 1986–96.

36. Caruso-Herman, "Concerns for the dying patient and family," pp. 120–23; Kelner, "Activists and delegators," pp. 537–45.

37. Rinaldi and Kearl, "The hospice farewell," pp. 283–300.

38. M. A. Mesler, "The philosophy and practice of patient control in hospice: The dynamics of autonomy versus paternalism," *Omega* 30, no. 3 (1995): 173–89.

39. Caruso-Herman, "Concerns for the dying patient and family," pp. 120–23; P. M. Koop and V. Strang, "Predictors of bereavement outcomes in families of patients with cancer: A literature review," *Canadian J Nurs Res* 29, no. 4 (1997): 33–50.

40. J. M. Brant, "The art of palliative care: Living with hope, dying with dignity," *Onc Nurs Forum* 25, no. 6 (1998): 995–1004.

41. C. Seale, J. Addington-Hall, and M. McCarthy, "Awareness of dying: Prevalence, causes, and consequences," *Social Science and Medicine* 45, no. 3 (1997): 477–84.

42. Brant, "The art of palliative care," pp. 995–1004.

43. Schultz and Hanusa, "Experimental social gerontology," pp. 30–46.

44. C. Campbell, "Suffering, compassion, and dignity in dying," *Duquesne Law Review* 35, no. 109 (1996): 33–50.

45. Byock, *Dying Well*.

46. Paton, "The sacred circle," pp. 52–56.

47. B. Moyer, *Healing and the Mind* (New York: Doubleday, 1993).

48. Thompson, "The future of death," pp. 175–80.

16

IN SEARCH OF A GOOD DEATH
Observations of Patients, Families, and Providers

Karen E. Steinhauser, Elizabeth C. Clipp, Maya McNeilly, Nicholas A. Christakis, Lauren M. McIntyre, and James A. Tulsky

Professional organizations and the public have recently made care of the dying a national priority.[1] Despite this, however, we remain confused about what constitutes a good death.[2] Some patients with terminal illnesses choose to leave the conventional medical setting and receive hospice care in their home, surrounded by family. Others seek experimental chemotherapy in an intensive care unit. In each of these vastly different scenarios, the perception of the quality of death is constructed by family, friends, and healthcare providers, not solely by the dying person. However, little empirical evidence exists to document these varied perspectives.[3]

We conducted this study to describe the attributes of a good death, as understood by various participants in end-of-life care. To evaluate the relative importance of these attributes, we compared the perspectives of different groups of persons who had experienced death in their personal or professional lives.

Reprinted from *Annals of Internal Medicine* 132 (2000): 825–32.

METHODS

DESIGN

We used focus groups and in-depth interviews to identify the attributes of a good death. These qualitative methods, which are common in exploratory studies, generate hypotheses and provide rich descriptive information about a phenomenon.[4] Researchers do not impose theoretical assumptions a priori but instead let participants frame questions from the "ground up."

PARTICIPANTS

Over a four-month period, we convened twelve focus groups, each of which had an average of six participants. A full spectrum of persons involved with end-of-life care—physicians, nurses, social workers, chaplains, hospice volunteers, patients, and recently bereaved family members—were included (see table 1).[5] Groups were stratified by role. Participants were recruited from Duke University Medical Center, Durham Veterans Affairs Medical Center, and a local community hospice in Durham, North Carolina. Nonphysician providers were recruited from convenience samples generated by e-mail and departmental advertising. Physicians were recruited from the attending staff of the Duke University Medical Center, Department of Medicine. We stratified physicians by level of appointment (assistant, associate, or full professor), randomized the lists, and recruited potential participants in order, ensuring that the final group represented each career level. Patients were recruited by telephone from an ethnically stratified sample enrolled in oncology and HIV clinics. Family members were recruited from a stratified random sample of recently bereaved relatives of Veterans Affairs patients who had died six months to one year earlier. For each group, we continued to call potential participants until we obtained six to eight participants per group.

Table 1. Focus Group Composition*

Participants	Group	Participants	Source
		n	
Nurses	3	27	VA Medical Center, Duke University Medical Center, community hospice
Social workers	2	10	VA Medical Center, Duke University Medical Center
Chaplains	1	6	VA Medical Center, Duke University Medical Center
Hospice volunteers	1	8	Community hospice
Physicians	1	6	VA Medical Center, Duke University Medical Center
Patients	3	14	VA Medical Center oncology and AIDS clinics
Bereaved family members[†]	1	4	Decedents of VA Medical Center

*VA = Veterans Affairs.
†The family focus group data were supplemented by data from hospice volunteers, most of whom were recently bereaved family members.

We conducted separate groups for African American and white patients, with trained facilitators from the respective ethnic groups. Participants were compensated for their time. The institutional review boards of the Durham Veterans Affairs Medical Center and the Duke University Medical Center approved the study.

DATA COLLECTION

We asked focus group participants to discuss their experiences with the deaths of family members, friends, or patients and to reflect on what made those deaths good or bad. When necessary, we asked probing questions to clarify a comment or obtain more detail.

We took several steps to ensure reliability and validity, which are often called "exhaustiveness" and "trustworthiness" in qualitative research.[6] First, we conducted focus groups until the same themes were repeated and no new themes emerged. Theme exhaustiveness is reached when similar themes are generated by participants from very different social backgrounds. Next, after repeatedly analyzing focus group transcripts, we conducted in-depth interviews with two members from each group—the most and least talkative participants. The most talkative participants were usually willing to provide information; the least talkative participants were interviewed to elicit possible silent but dissenting viewpoints. No new themes emerged through these interviews, thereby confirming exhaustiveness. The interviewees were presented with our analyses and were asked to evaluate our interpretations. Trustworthiness is noted when participants respond affirmatively to researchers' interpretations.[7]

STATISTICAL ANALYSIS

Focus groups and interviews were audiotaped and transcribed. We did not use quantitative methods of inter-rater agreement. Instead, we followed a grounded theory approach with a "constant comparisons" method and its related open and axial coding techniques.[8] During open coding, four investigators independently read an example of a transcript and analyzed it for common and recurrent themes pertaining to qualities of a good death. These summaries were compared for theme agreement and disagreement. One coder used qualitative software (NUDIST, Scolari Sage Publications Software, Thousand Oaks, California) to apply the coding scheme to the remaining transcripts. Throughout the coding process, all four investigators reviewed theme exemplars as a check on coding validity. During axial coding, the investigators developed further conceptual domains by comparing themes within and between transcripts.[9] After identifying more than seventy attributes, we collapsed the full list into six broad domains. Although the six themes are presented as conceptually distinct, attributes overlapped between domains. For example, attention to spiritual concerns may be primarily associated with a process of "completion" but may also affect patients' physical pain.

The illustrative quotes have been edited for ease of reading. We did not make any substantive changes but deleted repeated words and corrected grammatical inconsistencies that are common in spoken language.

RESULTS

Focus group participants ranged in age from twenty-six to seventy-seven years (mean age, forty-seven years) (see table 2). Sixty-four percent were women, 70 percent were white, and 28 percent were African American. Most (61 percent) of the sample was Protestant, 18 percent was Roman Catholic, and 8 percent identified themselves as Jewish. Six themes emerged: pain and symptom management, clear decision making, preparation for death, completion, contributing to others, and affirmation of the whole person (see table 3).

PAIN AND SYMPTOM MANAGEMENT

Many focus group participants feared dying in pain. Portrayals of bad deaths usually mentioned inadequate analgesia during cure-directed therapies that were perceived as too aggressive. One nurse, discussing a patient, said:

> His disease was very widespread. One of the interns or residents said, "We don't want you on morphine. You're going to get addicted." I said, "You must be joking. This guy is having pain, and he's not going to make it out of the hospital." He stayed on the surgical service and he died in 4 days, in pain.

Participants were concerned with both current pain control and control of future symptoms. Intrusive thoughts of break-through pain or extreme shortness of breath produced anxiety that could be relieved with appropriate reassurance. One man with

Table 2. Characteristics of Focus Group Participants*

Characteristic	Value
Age range, y	26–77
Mean age, y	46.8
Sex, %	
Male	36
Female	64
Ethnicity, %	
African American	28
Asian American	3
White	70
Religious affiliation, %	
Protestant	61
Roman Catholic	18
Jewish	8
Other	3
No affiliation	11
Recruitment source, %	
Veterans Affairs Medical Center	57
Duke University Medical Center	24
Community hospice	19

*Seventy-five persons participated. Values in some categories do not sum to 100 percent because of rounding.

AIDS said, "I don't want to be in pain, and I've discussed it with my doctor. He said, 'Oh, don't worry about pain. We'll put you on a morphine drip.' That sort of eased my mind."

CLEAR DECISION MAKING

Participants stated that fear of pain and inadequate symptom management could be reduced through communication and clear decision making with physicians. Patients felt empowered by participating in treatment decisions. One patient said:

This is *my* medical problem. Sometimes I don't want to stay on the rigid schedule, and he [the physician] would say, "I would

Table 3. Components of a Good Death

Pain and symptom management
Clear decision making
Preparation for death
Completion
Contributing to others
Affirmation of the whole person

like for you to stay on that, but you are the manager of your ship. You decide how fast you want to paddle, if you want to go backwards, sideways, or make a 360° turn."

Alternately, descriptions of bad deaths frequently included scenarios in which treatment preferences were unclear. Patients felt disregarded, family members felt perplexed and concerned about suffering, and providers felt out of control and feared that they were not providing good care. Decisions that had not previously been discussed usually had to be made during a crisis, when emotional reserves were already low.

One social worker, speaking about her mother, said:

I had never talked to her about end-of-life issues. I'm trying to communicate with my family over the phone. "What do we do? She's intubated, her labs are worse." The doctor said, "We really don't think that she's going to make it, and we have to consider withdrawing life support." I said, "I'm sorry, but that's not a decision I can make."

One physician spoke about the anticipatory conversations she usually had with patients who had advanced disease, using one particular patient as an example:

This person had mets everywhere. I explained to him, "There's nothing that's going to bring your bones back. In this situation, somebody would do CPR [cardiopulmonary resuscitation]. That involves pumping on your chest, and it would likely fracture your bones." I was very simple about it. I said, "The alternative, which I would recommend, is we make sure we give you enough pain medication that you will not suffer." I find that the more up-front I am, most people are appreciative of that.

PREPARATION FOR DEATH

Participants voiced a need for greater preparation for the end of life. Patients usually wanted to know what they could expect during the course of their illness and wanted to plan for the events that would follow their deaths. One patient said, "I have my will written out, who I want invited to the funeral. I have my obituary. That gives me a sense of completion that I don't have to put that burden on someone else. It's to prepare myself for it."

Family members felt a need to learn about the physical and psychosocial changes that would occur as death approached. Participants spoke of scenarios in which a lack of preparation adversely affected patient care. One nurse said:

> I can't tell you how many times, working in the emergency room, [that I saw] families [take a patient home]; this patient was going to die at home. And, when the last breath came, the families panicked. They brought the patient into the emergency room and went through the whole process [resuscitation]. Preparing the family, assessing what they actually know, and figuring out what you have to teach them is essential.

Finally, the most experienced nonphysician providers spoke about the importance of exploring one's own feelings about death and the ways in which these feelings influence the ability to care for terminally ill patients. One nurse said:

> When I was in nursing school, my older sister was killed in a car accident. I never had to think about death before that. It sent me on a personal quest. I developed a comfort with it that sometimes made it very frustrating to work with people who didn't have

that understanding, who still looked at death as the enemy. You all know which attendings can and can't go in and talk to the patients because it's too uncomfortable.

Most of the personal preparation described by healthcare providers had occurred individually, outside the context of their formal training. Only one physician in our study had received residency training in palliative medicine.

COMPLETION

Participants confirmed the deep importance of spirituality or meaningfulness at the end of life. Completion includes not only faith issues but also life review, resolving conflicts, spending time with family and friends, and saying good-bye. A family member of a recently deceased patient recalled the following:

He got home, and they got him out of the ambulance. I remember him saying, "Oh, can I wait just a minute, to remember the sunshine." This for somebody who hadn't seen the sun in. . . . It was almost like we had a party that evening. Everybody was there, and we sang songs. He died that night, at home, and everybody was there.

In Western culture, completion may be primarily a process of individual life review that is subsequently shared with family and friends. For patients from other cultures, completion may be more explicitly communal and may involve rituals that are important to the family during the dying process and after death. A nurse described her experiences with the family of one such patient:

They asked to bring in their religious representative. It was important to them that the patient be completely bathed [both] as she was dying as well as when she was dead. I had some weird looks from physicians who were saying, "You're wasting your time. This wasn't an effective intervention." But it was, because when all was said and done, they [the family] had accepted it.

Issues of faith were often mentioned as integral to overall healing at the end of life and frequently became more important as the patient declined physically. However, we also heard that such issues are highly individualistic and that cues about their particular expression must be taken from the patient.

CONTRIBUTING TO OTHERS

Several focus groups mentioned the importance of allowing terminally ill persons to contribute to the well-being of others. A hospice volunteer told the following story:

> They [patients] have the ability to help someone else through me. One fellow liked to go out for rides. He couldn't walk around very well, but he invited another patient to come out. She was very debilitated, too. So, the three of us would drive around the community. As debilitated as some patients get, they're still capable of helping someone else or making someone else laugh.

Contributions can take the form of gifts, time, or knowledge. As death approaches, many patients reflect on their successes and failures and discover that personal relationships outweigh professional or monetary gains. They are anxious to share that understanding with others. One family member said, "I guess it was really poignant for me when a nurse or new resident came into his room, and the first thing he'd say would be, 'Take care of your wife' or 'Take care of your husband. Spend time with your children.' He wanted to make sure he imparted that there's a purpose for life."

AFFIRMATION OF THE WHOLE PERSON

Participants repeatedly declared the importance of affirming the patient as a unique and whole person. Patients appreciated empathic healthcare providers. One patient said of his caretakers, "There's no question that they make me feel I can't ask." Family members were comforted by and spoke with great respect about those who did not treat their loved ones as a "disease" but understood them in the context of their lives, values, and preferences. One family member related the following:

> The residents always approached my father as if he was a person and there weren't any divisions between them. They didn't come in and say, "I'm Doctor so and so." There wasn't any kind of separation or aloofness. They would sit right on his bed, hold his hand, talk about their families, his family, golf, and sports.

Healthcare providers' descriptions of good deaths also focused on their personal relationships with patients and families. They were touched by the fact that these relationships were present even in the most dire medical crises. One physician told the following story about a patient:

> That last day I saw him in the emergency room, he was looking at me with those roving eyes and gasping for breath. I leaned over him and stroked his hair. He looked at me and said, "How's that new house of yours?" I said, "I'm not really moved in." And he said, "You make sure you decorate it nicely." It was a very personal interchange. He was dying, and his last interaction with me was as a person, not as a doctor.

DISTINCTIONS IN PERSPECTIVES OF A GOOD DEATH

These six themes reflect the common ground shared by participants. However, we also saw differences between groups. Social

and professional roles substantially shaped the views of our dis-
cussants. In fact, professional role distinctions were more pro-
nounced than sex or ethnic differences. For example, all social
workers spoke from a case management perspective and were
highly attuned to the needs of the family as the unit of care. Chaplains eloquently discussed ethical issues and were the only group
to relay the tension between individual and community rights.
Family members spoke from the unique role of both patient advocate and recipient of care. All six themes were present in patient,
family, and nonphysician healthcare provider focus groups. In
contrast, physicians' discussions were uniformly more medical in
nature, and no physicians spoke of "contributing to others." One
physician made a brief comment about completion, but other
members of the group did not expand on it.

DISCUSSION

Although death is a rite of passage in which we will all participate—as family member, provider, or, eventually, patient—we
understand little of what is valued at the end of life. Our study
confirmed the importance of four themes found in the palliative
care literature: pain and symptom management, clear decision
making, preparation for death, and completion. Two new themes,
contributing to others and affirmation of the whole person, were
unexpected and add to our understanding.

Every provider group offered regret-filled stories of patients
who died in pain. Such findings are concordant with studies
showing that 40 percent to 70 percent of Americans have substantial pain in the last days of their lives.[10] Concern about undertreatment of pain is consistent across surveys of physicians, nurses, and
recently bereaved family members.[11] Our study also revealed a
new dimension to this theme: anticipatory fears about pain and
symptom control. Many dying persons are terrified of waking in

the middle of the night with intense pain or air hunger. For them, a good death includes providers who anticipate these fears.

Providers and families in our study also identified the need for improved communication and clear decision making and feared entering a medical crisis without knowledge of patient preferences. Despite the recent attention devoted to advance care planning, this remains a source of great consternation.[12] Medicine will never remove all uncertainty from the decision-making process.[13] However, if values and preferences are clarified, tolerance for that uncertainty may increase.

Focus group members were concerned about our society's tendency to deny death and demanded greater preparation for dying. We heard many examples in which providers avoided end-of-life discussions because they did not want to remove hope. However, patients and families feared bad dying more than death. Bad dying was characterized by lack of opportunity to plan ahead, arrange personal affairs, decrease family burden, or say good-bye. For dying patients and their families, preparation does not preclude hope; it merely frames it. After a new diagnosis, patients usually hope for a cure. However, they also hope for lack of pain, lucidity, good quality of life, and a physician who is committed to being with them throughout the care process.

We heard extensive discussion of the need for "completion," a process involving meaningful time with family and close friends and attention to religious or spiritual beliefs. Terminally ill patients are often able to view their current experience as part of a broader life course trajectory. This may explain why they often rate their quality of life higher than observers, who often do not give appropriate weight to patients' emotional and spiritual development during the dying process.[14] Traditional measures used to assess end-of-life quality do not usually account for this growth potential.[15]

Our study introduced two novel components of a good death. First, a surprising number of participants spoke of the importance of terminally ill patients' contributions to the well-being of others.

We fully expected to find that dying patients needed care, but we did not consider the extent to which they also needed to reciprocate. Social psychologists describe this need for "generativity" as one of the great emotional tasks of human development, particularly during later life.[16] Dying patients need to participate in the same human interactions that are important throughout all of life. Second, focus group participants continually discussed the need to appreciate patients as unique and "whole persons," not only as "diseases" or cases. We were struck by the very personal language of this theme and by participants' desire to simply be known.

These six themes add to our understanding of what constitutes a good death and also generate hypotheses that have implications for both medical education and clinical practice. The culture of death changed dramatically during the twentieth century. When people died primarily at home, family, community, and clergy assumed responsibility. As the location of death shifted to the hospital, physicians became the gatekeepers.[17] As a result, death is now viewed through the lens of biomedical explanation and is primarily defined as a physiologic event.[18] Most medical education and training reinforces this framework.

However, a strictly biomedical perspective is incomplete. For most persons involved with care at the end of life, death is infused with broader meaning and is considered a natural part of life, not a failure of technology. All focus groups, except physicians, spoke extensively about the need for life review and subsequent completion. This is not to suggest that these themes are unimportant to physicians; rather, they are not a usual focus of treatment. It may be useful to recognize that for most patients and families who are confronting death and dying, psychosocial and spiritual issues are as important as physiologic concerns. Patients and families want relationships with healthcare providers that affirm this more encompassing view.

In an economic environment that substantially limits physicians' time, developing such relationships may seem unrealistic.

However, in a previous study, we noted that the median time for advance directive discussions is less than ten minutes, with no apparent correlation between length of discussion and discussion quality.[19] Furthermore, an initial investment of time may improve the patient-physician relationship and save time in future conversations. Time may also be used more efficiently if providers have an a priori list of themes to touch on, such as the six discussed here.

There is no single formula for a good death. Many participants cautioned healthcare providers against implying, "You're not dying the right way because you're not dying the way we think you should." As one author has written, people die "in character."[20] Professional providers who meet a dying patient for the first time are at a disadvantage because they catch only a cross-sectional glimpse of the lifetime of experiences that are shaping the dying process. Our data suggest that the quality of dying is related to acknowledgment of that lifetime context.

We heard many stories of healthcare providers' discomfort with death and dying. Whether such discomfort is caused by feelings of failure, a desire for professional distance, or inexperience, it can adversely affect care. Delivering bad news or discussing other end-of-life issues is a skill that is rarely natural; like other procedures, it must be learned.[21] Furthermore, providers must be able to acknowledge and process the feelings that arise when caring for dying patients.[22] Programs designed to facilitate this process are now common in police departments and crisis intervention programs, two occupational settings in which trauma and death are always present.[23] However, such programs have not yet become a usual part of medical training or practice.

Physicians should also be reminded that they are not alone when caring for dying patients; many other healthcare providers (nurses, social workers, and chaplains) are available for comprehensive care. For example, physicians may ask a screening question (such as "What role does faith or spirituality play in your life?") that displays awareness of these important aspects. Physicians can then ask whether the patient would like to speak in greater depth with a chaplain. Although physicians may not be responsible for resolving the psychosocial and spiritual needs of patients, acknowledging the presence and complexity of these needs is a way of actively affirming the whole person.

Our study has several limitations. Most patients were recruited from a Veterans Affairs medical center, and therefore our findings may not be generalizable to other groups. Although our patients were mostly men, they represented a broad range of ages, educational levels, and socioeconomic backgrounds. Many also received care in the private sector, and their comments reflected experiences in many settings. Family focus group members were also recruited from the Veterans Affairs system. However, we collected extensive discussions of family perspectives during discussions with the hospice volunteer group and follow-up interviews with patients. Discussions were limited to deaths from chronic illness and did not include deaths caused by accident or trauma. However, participants described deaths that had occurred in hospices, hospitals, and at home. Good and bad deaths occurred in all settings.

Our study has implications for clinicians, educators, and researchers. Although there is no "right" way to die, the six themes identified here provide an initial framework for addressing topics that are important to patients and families. In addition, biomedical aspects of end-of-life care are crucial but merely provide a point of departure toward a good death. When physical symptoms are properly palliated, patients and families may have the opportunity to address the critical psychosocial and spiritual issues they face at the end of life.

NOTES

1. Council on Scientific Affairs, "Good care of the dying patient," *JAMA* 275 (1996): 474–78; *Patient Self-Determination Act of 1990, Omnibus Budget Reconciliation Act* (OBRA), Public Law 101–508; M. J. Field and

C. K. Cassel, *Approaching Death: Improving Care at the End of Life* (Washington, D.C.: National Academy Press, 1997); B. Lo and L. Snyder, "Care at the end of life: Guiding practice where there are no easy answers," *Ann Intern Med* 130 (1997): 722–24; I. Byock, *Dying Well: The Prospect for Growth at the End of Life* (New York: Riverhead Books, 1997); Veterans Health Administration Directive, policy on implementation of hospice program, 1990; *Veterans' Health Care Eligibility Reform Act of 1996*, House Resolution 3118, section 341, 1990.

2. P. Aries, *The Hour of Our Death* (New York: Alfred A. Knopf, 1980).

3. F. J. Fowler, K. M. Coppola, and J. M. Teno, "Methodological challenges for measuring care at the end of life," *J Pain & Sympt Mgmt* 17 (1999): 114–19; P. A. Singer, D. K. Martin, and M. Kelner, "Quality end-of-life care: Patients' perspectives," *JAMA* 281 (1999): 163–68.

4. J. Corbin and A. Strauss, *Basics of Qualitative Research* (Thousand Oaks, Calif.: Sage, 1990); R. Krueger, *Focus Groups: A Practical Guide for Applied Research*, 2d ed. (Thousand Oaks, Calif.: Sage, 1994); P. Stern, "Using grounded theory method in nursing research," in *Qualitative Research Methods in Nursing*, ed. M. M. Leninger (Orlando, Fla.: Grune and Stratton, 1985).

5. Krueger, *Focus Groups*.

6. Corbin and Strauss, *Basics of Qualitative Research*.

7. Krueger, *Focus Groups*.

8. Singer, Martin, and Kelner, "Quality end-of-life care," pp. 163–68; Corbin and Strauss, *Basics of Qualitative Research*.

9. Corbin and Strauss, *Basics of Qualitative Research*.

10. A controlled trial to improve care for seriously ill hospitalized patients. SUPPORT Principal Investigators, "The study to understand prognoses and preferences for outcomes and risks of treatments (SUPPORT)," *JAMA* 274 (1995): 1591–98.

11. Singer, Martin, and Kelner, "Quality end-of-life care," pp. 163–68; M. Z. Solomon, "The enormity of the task: SUPPORT and changing practice," *Hastings Center Report* 25 (1995): 528–32; L. C. Hanson, M. Danis, and J. Garrett, "What is wrong with end-of-life care? Opinions of bereaved family members," *J Am Geriatr Soc* 45 (1997): 1339–44.

12. *Patient Self-Determination Act of 1990*; L. L. Emanuel et al., "Advance directives for medical care—a case for greater use," *N Engl J Med* 324 (1991): 889–95; L. L. Emanuel et al., "Advance care planning as a

process: Structuring the discussions in practice," *J Am Geriatr Soc* 43 (1995): 440–46.

13. N. A. Christakis, *Death Foretold: Prophecy and Prognosis in Medical Care* (Chicago: University of Chicago Press, 1999).

14. S. R. Cohen et al., "The McGill quality of life questionnaire: A measure of quality of life appropriate for people with advanced disease: A preliminary study of validity and acceptability," *Palliat Med* 9 (1995): 207–19; S. R. Cohen and B. M. Mount, "Quality of life in terminal illness: Defining and measuring subjective well-being in the dying," *J Palliat Care* 8 (1992) 40–45; E. C. Clipp and L. K. George, "Patients with cancer and their spouse caregivers: Perceptions of the illness experience," *Cancer* 69 (1992): 1074–79; M. Fowlie, J. Berkely, and I. Dingwall-Fordyce, "Quality of life in advanced cancer: The benefits of asking the patient," *Palliat Med* 3 (1989): 55–59; M. A. Sprangers and N. K. Aaronson, "The role of health-care providers and significant others in evaluating the quality of life of patients with chronic disease: A review," *J Clin Epidemiol* 45 (1992): 743–60.

15. Cohen et al., "The McGill quality of life questionnaire," pp. 207–19.

16. E. H. Erikson, *The Life Cycle Completed: A Review* (New York: W. W. Norton, 1982).

17. S. R. Kaufman, "Intensive care, old age, and the problem of death in America," *Gerontologist* 38 (1998): 715–25; P. Starr, *The Social Transformation of American Medicine* (Cambridge: Harvard University Press, 1982).

18. Kaufman, "Intensive care, old age, and the problem of death in America," pp. 715–25; M. Foucault, *The Birth of the Clinic: An Archeology of Medical Perception* (New York: Pantheon Books, 1973).

19. J. A. Tulsky, M. A. Chesney, and B. Lo, "How do medical residents discuss resuscitation with patients?" *J Gen Intern Med* 10 (1995): 436–42; J. A. Tulsky et al., "Opening the black box: How do physicians communicate about advance directives?" *Ann Intern Med* 129 (1998): 441–49.

20. T. R. McCormick and B. J. Conley, "Patients' perspectives on dying and on the care of dying patients," *West J Med* 163 (1995): 236–43.

21. J. Tulsky, M. Chesney, and B. Lo, "See one, do one, teach one? House staff experience discussing do-not-resuscitate orders," *Arch Intern Med* 156 (1996): 1258–59.

22. B. Lo, T. Quill, and J. Tulsky, "Discussing palliative care with

patients, ACP-ASIM End-of-Life Care Consensus Panel, American College of Physicians–American Society of Internal Medicine," *Ann Intern Med* 130 (1999): 744–49.

23. K. Armstrong et al., "Debriefing of American Red Cross personnel: Pilot study on participants' evaluations and case examples from the 1994 Los Angeles earthquake relief operation," *Soc Work Health Care* 27 (1998): 33–50; P. A. Rosebush, "Psychological intervention with military personnel in Rwanda," *Military Med* 163 (1998): 559–63; J. Cudmore, "Preventing post-traumatic stress disorder in accident and emergency nursing: A review of the literature," *Nurs Crit Care* 1 (1996): 120–26.

17

THE JEWISH PATIENT AND TERMINAL DEHYDRATION
A Hospice Ethical Dilemma

Janet Bodell and Marie-Ange Weng

INTRODUCTION

Within the pluralistic milieu of the United States, the hospice industry actively seeks to provide culturally competent care to the terminally ill. Since the "desire to put those people who are different from oneself into categories . . . leads to depersonalization,"[1] the challenge for hospice nurses in caring for the Jewish patient is complex, especially when presented with the issue of terminal dehydration. For the Jewish patient, as part of an intensely life-affirming culture, terminal dehydration presents an ethical dilemma for end-of-life care. The hospice nurse must consider the Jewish historical, cultural, and theological viewpoints as related to the individual patient when assisting the patient and his or her family in making or rejecting this choice.

Reprinted from *American Journal of Hospice & Palliative Care* 17, no. 3 (May/June 2000): 185–88.

PERSPECTIVES OF THE JEWISH COMMUNITY

IN THE UNITED STATES

Historically, the Jews learned to carry on their traditions simply by living their lives in community, taking care of their own. "It doesn't happen that way anymore. Jewish families are scattered and the community is dispersed."[2] Thus, it is probable to anticipate caring for a Jewish person within the secular hospice industry.

Also, depending upon the particular movement to which a Jew might belong (Orthodox, Conservative, Reform, Reconstructionist), not all adherents of the particular religious communities necessarily stick to all the rules and customs. "The non-Orthodox Jews ... tend to view *halachah* (traditional Jewish law) as a reference point and guide rather than mandate."[3] Then, Neuberger indicates:

> Large numbers of Jews everywhere regard themselves as Jewish by peoplehood rather than by religion. . . . In addition, the life-affirming strand in Judaism is very strong, even amongst those who are disaffected from the religion itself.[4]

Dennis relates that, at least in the United States, "Jewishness plays perhaps a bigger role in their lives than does religion."[5]

WITHHOLDING OR WITHDRAWING

Terminal dehydration, i.e., withholding or withdrawing food and fluid as a means to allow a terminally ill patient to die, has particular aversion for the Jewish population because of the value Jews give to life and to food as a life-sustaining, healing, and comforting agent; the fine line between what is life sustaining versus what is death prolonging; and, last, the conflicting viewpoints within the various Jewish sects.

Because of the historical experience of starvation under impoverished conditions in Eastern European ghettos and in the concentration camps of Nazi Germany, food is closely associated with the value of life for most Jews.[6] Also, from the time of the "12th century philosopher-physician, Moses Ben Maimon (Maimonides) . . . chicken soup . . . has achieved the status of a standing joke among Jews[7] as a healing agent. "Food [in general] plays a large part in the folk religion of Judaism."[8]

Second, the Torah commands Jews to "choose life."[9] It may be difficult to ascertain what is life sustaining versus that which may be death prolonging. "The Jewish law states that 'it is permitted to remove the impediment to dying,' " but, on the other hand, it speaks in terms of duty[10] and here there is a duty to live if at all possible.

Diamant gives an example of just how important it is for Jews to sustain life:

> The religious principle of preserving human life (p'kuach nefesh) is considered a primary mandate. A Jew may break every Jewish law—eat pork, work on the Sabbath—if it might save a life or promote the healing of someone who is ill.[11]

Gordon contrasts the biomedical ethicist who considers intravenous therapy and tube feedings to be forms of medical treatment (medicine) with the Jewish position that is unclear and much debated within and among the various sects. Some rabbinical authorities distinguish between "nutrition and hydration" that is required by all living beings and "medicine."[12] There is a Jewish saying, stated a rabbinical student, "If you have two Jews debating an issue, you will end up with three opinions!" "Those who take their Jewish heritage seriously will continue to disagree with one another."[13]

THE JEWISH PATIENT WITHIN THE U.S. HOSPICE INDUSTRY

JEWISH VIEW OF DEATH

"The [Jewish] tradition views death as a part of life and teaches that there is 'a time to die.' "[14] However, when is a person considered to be dying and what does the Jewish law teach about this? Gordon states:

> The law concerning a *goses* [dying person], defined by the rabbis as "one who is within three days of death," is that one may not do anything to shorten the person's life, even to relieve his or her suffering.[15]

The dilemma of withdrawing food and fluid becomes tied into the limited time frame of three days before death to say that one is a "dying person." Then, Hall, an attorney, counsels that "more than the emotional reaction to withholding food and fluid . . . removing [them] will certainly cause death."[16] In Judaism, there is "less concern with belief than with action or *mitzvah* that means "commandment" or "sacred obligation."[17] Thus, even for the terminally ill patient who is not yet considered a *goses* by Jewish law, that commandment is to *live* every moment to the fullest, which includes taking in food and fluid naturally or, in many cases, artificially.

Another factor in the dilemma of whether to withhold or withdraw food and fluid is the Jewish "compulsive shying-away from discussion [of death] . . . in fact [Jews are] deathly afraid of death."[18] This denial of death, at times, or unwillingness to discuss death, for whatever reason, may deter the terminally ill person from being identified as a *goses*. Even medical ethicists admit that the ideal of assessing those who are irreversibly dying "is difficult to satisfy . . . in making judgments of futility,"[19] meaning that the diagnosis of terminal system failure is not always that clear. The value judgment of what life means for the Jewish patient, and also "what is worth the effort," may only be judged by the Jewish patient himself or herself and the patient's family if he or she is unable to make the decision.

MISTRUST

It is a fact that many Jews mistrust the U.S. hospice industry, basically on two religious-cultural issues. "First, Jews commonly perceive that hospice is a Christian movement. . . . Second . . . American Jewry's culturally based anxiety around death issues,"[20] as previously discussed.

For Jews, perceiving hospice as a "Christian" movement might bring thoughts of fear, abandonment, and desecration of the body. *Fear* is because of past experiences with anti-Semitism; *abandonment* is because the Jewish patient and family might not be aware that hospice would allow the *mitzvah* of *"bikkur holim,"*[21] i.e., being present continuously at the bedside of the terminally ill person; *desecration of the body* is because the Jewish laws regarding the care of the body at the time of death and after death are quite explicit and very different from Christian ways. With the perception of hospice as Christian, questions might arise such as, "Would a Christian be sensitive to Jewish ways?" "Would I be able to have my Jewish customs and traditions honored?" This doubt is often present in the Jewish patient and family, even though the general hospice industry is quite transculturally oriented and, for the most part, secular.

Also, the locus of time concept is very different for a terminally ill Jewish patient, as compared to a Christian patient. If Jews perceived that only the Christian concept of looking forward to the afterlife and giving one's life over to a loving, personal Lord [God] were maintained in hospice care, the Jew's own time concept of the *here and now* might be thought to be misunderstood or neglected. Although many Jews believe in an afterlife, they do not generally think about what may happen after death, nor do they dwell on it. "A life well lived, rather than a 'good death' is the primary preoccupation for the Jew of faith."[22] "Judaism's relative indifference to the afterlife is apparent in the [Jewish] laws and customs that surround death."[23]

FAMILY AND COMMUNITY

Relationship is a key concept in Jewish spirituality.[24] Important to the terminally ill Jewish patient is the inclusion of family and often those from his/her Jewish community. Rabbi Dennis comments, using the concept "good death" as an analogy:

> A "good death" [for Jews is] . . . one in which suffering is minimized; their value is affirmed by family, friends, and community; they are assured of continued remembrance by the community of faith; and they have confidence that all of their life before that moment had meaning.[25]

TRANSCULTURAL, ETHICAL, AND LEGAL CONSIDERATIONS

In the United States, there are underlying "values implicit in ethics and law about dying and death."[26] Nurses see these values reflected in their professional code of ethics, based on the Hippocratic perspective. The number one principle of this perspective says, "do no harm." Transcultural, ethical, and legal considerations regarding terminal dehydration (withholding and withdrawing food and fluid) when caring for the terminally ill Jewish patient within the general hospice industry must include the application of several ethical principles, namely, justice, autonomy, beneficence, and nonmaleficence.

JUSTICE

Justice, referring to the "value of fairness, requires treating all people . . . without bias."[27] It is vital that hospice personnel be aware that Jews are acutely cognizant of the fact that "[the Holocaust] started with the acceptance of the attitude . . . that there is such a thing as a life not worthy to be lived."[28] The principle of justice in this case says that such an attitude has no place in hospice toward any patient. The Jewish patient's individual needs and wishes must be considered by hospice personnel in light of this history of "horror" and all this may imply for a Jewish patient in a non-Jewish setting.

AUTONOMY

The ethical principle of autonomy relates to the "notion of self-determination. The notion of informed consent is the legal extension [of this principle]."[29] Advance directives, an ethical will, and collaboration with the patient and family in developing the nursing care plan are interventions to promote exercising the principle of autonomy for the Jewish patient. Rabbi Gordon counsels Jewish congregants:

> You can protect yourself from unwanted medical treatment when you are no longer competent by preparing advance directives. . . . Because no document can anticipate every possible medical event, you should also appoint someone as your *healthcare proxy* to make choices for you.[30]

Terminally ill Jewish patients should be counseled on the possibility of withholding or withdrawing food and fluid, so that they can make their wishes known in the advance directive and, more important, to their healthcare proxy to deal with any unexpected circumstances according to the wishes of the terminally ill patient.

An ethical will is a "time-honored Jewish custom of leaving a spiritual legacy to family and friends."[31] The patient desiring to do this may want help from a rabbi. An ethical will challenges the Jewish patient to name what is most important in his/her life and how he/she wishes to be remembered.[32] The ethical will is mentioned here because, in the event that food and fluid are withheld or withdrawn, the dying patient may want his or her family to have the written legacy that he or she valued life, but also did not seek to prolong death, according to the Jewish law.

Finally, applying the principle of autonomy entreats the hospice nurse to collaborate with the Jewish patient and his or her family in developing the nursing care plan. Physical care, including the possibility of withholding or withdrawing food and fluid, must be discussed; emotional and psychological care, including support systems the patient already enjoys and support systems that hospice provides, if needed or desired; and, last, spiritual care, as to whom a Jewish patient may wish to provide this care. For a religious or a nonreligious Jew, inform the patient that hospice provides spiritual care to patients within the concept that says all patients are spiritual, while some are religious and some are not. Hospice spiritual care is nonproselytizing and refers to a compassionate and empathetic *presence* of one human being to another. This care may provide much comfort to the Jewish patient and family at the time the decision to withhold or withdraw food and fluid is considered.

BENEFICENCE AND NONMALEFICENCE

Finally, the principles of beneficence (doing good) and nonmaleficence (do no harm) may be applied to the care interventions for the Jewish patient and family when making the decision to choose or reject terminal dehydration for end-of-life care. "It is necessary to explore family caregiver perceptions of . . . terminal dehydration."[33] It may be beneficial to recount the Cox study, where:

Cox distinguished between the acute symptoms accompanying sudden fluid discontinuance in healthy adults from those symptoms that develop gradually during the process of natural death. Dr. Cox's opinion that terminal dehydration is not painful is based on observations of more than four thousand patients encountered.[34]

Also, counsel the patient and family that the hospice perspective of this intervention relates to the motive of keeping the patient comfortable and *not* to "kill the patient." Inform the patient and family of the time when a human body may no longer benefit from what should be beneficial, i.e., food and fluid. Actually, providing food and fluid might burden a patient, who, not being able to metabolize them at life's end, will be subjected to peripheral and pulmonary edema. Zerwekh[35] writes of "benefits" of terminal dehydration at the end of life. The benefits are fewer episodes of incontinence, fewer bouts of vomiting, and tubes or suctioning will not be necessary for decompression. One study she cites also points to a possible "anesthetic effect through blood chemistry changes."[36]

Frequent evaluation and reassessment of the terminally ill Jewish patient are imperative to apply the principle of nonmaleficence. Because life is so valued by Jews, making these choices regarding end-of-life issues, such as withdrawing or withholding food and fluid, attempting to know when life is not being sustained but death is being prolonged, can be painful for the Jewish family, as for any family. The hospice nurse must be informed of the clinical picture to relate this information in a sensitive and timely way, so that the Jewish patient (if possible) and family are able to make an informed choice according to their particular Jewish perspective.

CONCLUSION

Terminal dehydration may be a viable option for end-of-life care for the Jewish patient, provided that a delineative report of the patient's declining condition is given to the family (or healthcare proxy) if the patient is unable to speak for himself or herself. The hospice nurse should give detailed clinical signs, if possible, that further intervention, such as providing food or fluid, may actually prolong the dying process, which is against traditional Jewish law, and thus may help the family to make an informed choice. Also, it is imperative for the hospice nurse to be sensitive to the fact that terminal dehydration may present an ethical dilemma when caring for a terminally ill Jewish patient because of the often difficult decision of determining that a Jewish patient is within the three-day period before death to be considered a dying person (*goses*), when, according to Jewish law, an impediment may be removed. Last, the hospice nurse must develop a collaborative nursing care plan with supportive measures by using interventions that mark outcomes which apply the ethical principles of justice, autonomy, beneficence, and nonmaleficence.

NOTES

1. J. Neuberger, "Cultural issues in palliative care: Introduction," in *Oxford Textbook of Palliative Medicine*, 2d ed., ed. D. Doyle, G. W. C. Hands, and N. MacDonald (New York: Oxford University Press, 1998).

2. A. Diamant, *Saying Kaddish: How to Comfort the Dying, Bury the Dead, and Mourn as a Jew* (New York: Schocken Books, 1998).

3. Ibid.

4. Neuberger, "Cultural issues in palliative care."

5. G. Dennis, "Love is as strong as death: Meeting the pastoral needs of the Jewish hospice patient," *Am J Hosp & Palliat Care* 16, no. 4 (1999): 598–604.

6. Neuberger, "Cultural issues in palliative care."

7. Dennis, "Love is as strong as death," pp. 598–604.

8. Neuberger, "Cultural issues in palliative care."

9. H. L. Gordon, *Questions and Answers about Jewish Tradition and the Issues of Assisted Death* (New York: Union of American Hebrew Congregations, 1998).

10. Ibid.

11. Diamant, *Saying Kaddish.*

12. Gordon, *Questions and Answers about Jewish Tradition.*

13. Ibid.

14. Diamant, *Saying Kaddish.*

15. Gordon, *Questions and Answers about Jewish Tradition.*

16. J. K. Hall, *Nursing: Ethics and Law* (Philadephia: W. B. Saunders, 1996).

17. Diamant, *Saying Kaddish.*

18. M. Lamm, *The Jewish Way in Death and Mourning* (New York: Jonathan David Publishers, 1969).

19. T. L. Beauchamp and J. F. Childress, *Principles of Biomedical Ethics,* 4th ed. (New York: Oxford University Press, 1994).

20. Dennis, "Love is as strong as death," pp. 598–604.

21. Diamant, *Saying Kaddish.*

22. Dennis, "Love is as strong as death," pp. 598–604.

23. Diamant, *Saying Kaddish.*

24. Dennis, "Love is as strong as death," pp. 598–604.

25. Ibid.

26. J. K. Hall, *Nursing: Ethics and Law.*

27. Ibid.

28. Ibid.

29. C. J. Meares, "Terminal dehydration: A review," *Am J Hosp & Palliat Care* 11, no. 3 (1994): 10–14.

30. Gordon, *Questions and Answers about Jewish Tradition.*

31. Diamant, *Saying Kaddish.*

32. Ibid.

33. Meares, "Terminal dehydration," pp. 10–14.

34. Ibid.

35. J. V. Zerwekh, "Do dying patients really need IV fluids?" *Amer J Nurs* 97, no. 3 (1997): 28.

36. Ibid.

Part Four

LEGAL ISSUES
AT THE
END OF LIFE

18

AVOIDING FAMILY FEUDS
Responding to Surrogate Demands for Life-Sustaining Interventions

Ann Alpers and Bernard Lo

The laws and ethical guidelines governing decision making for incompetent patients evolved from controversies in which family members refused life-sustaining interventions.[1] These cases led to a consensus that advance directives to limit interventions should be respected and that a surrogate designated by the patient or specified by statute could refuse interventions, even when other relatives disagreed.[2] Surrogate decision-making statutes and ethical principles about respect for delegated autonomy promote an active role for family members or other surrogates in medical decisions for incompetent patients. Inviting surrogates to participate actively in medical decisions recognizes the importance of the patient's personal community and assures that decisions will reflect the patient's own preferences and values.

The standard approach to decisions for incompetent adults gives advance directives priority over a surrogate's substituted judgment, which in turn has priority over assessments of the

Reprinted from *Journal of Law, Medicine & Ethics* 27, no. 1 (spring 1999): 74–80, by permission of the American Society of Law, Medicine & Ethics. All rights reserved.

patient's best interests.[3] A patient may express advance directives by appointing a proxy, stating specific preferences, or articulating general values. We use case examples to illustrate the limitations of all three types of advance directives.

Another standard encourages patients to designate a single proxy and gives that individual priority over other friends and relatives. Such proxy designation makes particular sense for gay men with acquired immune deficiency syndrome, who want their partners or friends to make decisions for them.[4] A single designated surrogate can also resolve a case in which several relatives disagree.[5] However, our cases illustrate how surrogates often make decisions as members of a family unit whose relationships will continue after the patient's death.

The relationship between surrogates and physicians usually promotes good decision making for incompetent patients. However, conflicts can emerge when surrogates insist on interventions that physicians consider inappropriate for patients at the end of life.[6] These conflicts pit the ethical obligation to respect the patient's autonomy as delegated to the surrogate against the professional integrity of physicians and the well-being of the patient.

Professional integrity has garnered much less attention in the literature than the ethical values of autonomy and nonmaleficence. Nonetheless, professional integrity functions as an ethical principle that reflects the moral commitment physicians profess when they practice medicine.[7] Using examples like sexual contact between physicians and patients and euthanasia, Howard Brody emphasizes the importance of internal ethical standards to define medicine's legitimate practice, even when those standards are controversial or contradict the preferences of some individual physicians and patients.[8] Edmund Pellegrino argues that physicians are moral agents whose integrity must be respected by patients; neither the patient nor the physician "may impose his or her values on the other."[9] Tom Beauchamp and James Childress emphasize that integrity involves "being faithful to moral values and standing up in their defense when they are threatened or under attack."[10] Physician integrity includes an injunction not to perform interventions for which the predictable harms outweigh the potential benefits.[11] In other words, surrogates' choice, no matter how well intentioned, should not make physicians agents of harm. Hence, professional integrity can also be grounded on the ethical principle of nonmaleficence.

This article analyzes two cases that illustrate the conflicts between the ethical obligation to respect the autonomy delegated to surrogates and the ethical obligations to maintain professional integrity and refrain from harming patients. The scenarios are based on real cases that were referred to a hospital ethics committee (EC) as intractable disputes complicated by issues of politics, culture, and ethnicity. The cases show how standard ethical and legal approaches to incompetent patients may fail to resolve these conflicts. In the first case, the patient had given clear advance directives and had appointed a healthcare proxy. In the second, the patient had stated his general values and goals. He also had a legal surrogate—his wife. Nonetheless, conflict arose between these patients' surrogates and the medical teams. We discuss how physicians could ethically forgo interventions in such situations, despite surrogates' insistence on them. In the first instance, we argue that physicians have ethical obligations to clarify whether the current situation differs from what the patient envisaged when giving advance directives. In the second, we argue that physicians have ethical obligations to clarify how the patient himself would have defined his best interests when surrogates request interventions that cause considerable suffering to the patient but little medical benefit. Clarification here should be based on general advance directives. Such actions are dictated by both professional integrity and the principle of nonmaleficence. To carry out these responsibilities, physicians will need to have extensive discussions with the patient's surrogates and to negotiate with them to resolve differing notions of the patient's best interests.[12]

INTERPRETING ADVANCE DIRECTIVES IN AN UNANTICIPATED SITUATION

The patient in case 1 gave specific preferences about care, which he discussed extensively with his healthcare proxy and relatives.

CASE 1

Mr. A, a forty-two-year-old gay man with the human immuno-deficiency virus and cirrhosis from hepatitis C, was admitted for liver transplantation under an experimental protocol. He developed renal failure, adult respiratory distress syndrome, cachexia, encephalopathy, and repeated episodes of sepsis. He could not be weaned from a ventilator. To be a transplantation candidate, he needed to be off the ventilator, free of infection, and clinically stable.

Mr. A had chosen liver transplantation after extensive deliberation. He appointed his partner as his healthcare proxy. His brother, a critical care nurse with training in ethics, quit his job to nurse Mr. A. Mr. A had repeatedly said that he wanted aggressive care, no matter what the circumstances. The day before extubation was last attempted, he said he would rather be two weeks too late in turning off life support than two hours too early. He currently is unresponsive.

Because Mr. A is no longer a transplantation candidate, the medical staff raises the issue of forgoing life-sustaining interventions. The physicians believe that continued intensive care would only prolong his dying. The family (the patient's partner, brother, and mother) believes that the patient's stated wishes should be respected.

Once it became clear that Mr. A could not receive a transplant, his preference for aggressive treatment had to be interpreted in light of a different medical situation. The family, however, had promised him that they would do what he wanted and were reluctant to contradict his explicit preferences. The family had to confront the problem that advance directives cannot anticipate every situation. Mr. A's oral advance directive made requests for specific interventions so that he could receive a liver transplant. In essence, it provided anticipatory informed consent to the multitude of tests and treatments necessary to undergo transplantation and postoperative care. However, he never had the opportunity to clarify his preferences after it had been determined that he would not receive a transplant. Once transplantation was not an option, his advance directive no longer provided meaningful consent, because it was predicated on a clinical situation that was no longer accurate. The EC, when consulted, suggested that it was ethically appropriate for the family to contradict the patient's directive. In the EC's view, because the current situation fundamentally differed from what the patient understood when he stated his preferences in his advance directive, the specific decisions it contained no longer applied. A decision based on incorrect medical assumptions and facts could not reflect the patient's autonomous choice. Therefore, it was ethically acceptable for the family to diverge from Mr. A's specific directives to accommodate his new prognosis and medical options. Such discretion for surrogates is also justified because patients vary in how strictly they want surrogates to follow their directives. In one study, 31 percent of patients stated that they would give surrogates complete leeway to override their advance directives if it were in their best interests, while 39 percent stated they would give surrogates no leeway.[13]

But, what if the patient had insisted at the onset on maximal treatment, even if he did not receive a liver transplant? In other words, what if a patient intended an advance directive to apply to all possible scenarios, even if it only made sense to the physicians to apply it in limited medical circumstances? Such a directive would offer the opportunity for the patient and healthcare team to discuss in advance what the patient meant by "maximal treatment" and what goals of care the patient hoped to fulfill. Usually, the physician and patient can negotiate a mutually acceptable plan of care; however, if disagreements are irreconcilable, the doctor and patient may decide to terminate their relationship.[14] When rigorous outcomes studies yield good data on the efficacy of life-sustaining interventions, physicians are obligated by professional ethics to explain these limitations to patients. For example, if studies allow presumptive guidelines for limiting life-sustaining interventions in certain clinical situations to patients who have had bone marrow transplantation,[15] these guidelines should be explained to patients who are planning on undergoing this procedure. In this way, conflicting expectations for care can be addressed and negotiated before the procedure is carried out.

INTERPRETING A PATIENT'S GENERAL VALUES

A patient's general goals for medical care do not always predict preferences regarding specific interventions.[16] Case 2 shows the difficulty of applying a patient's general religious beliefs to decisions about specific medical interventions.

CASE 2

Bishop P is a sixty-year-old African American man who suffers from quadriplegia and persistent infections. He is the retired prelate of a Pentecostal church that emphasizes faith healing. One year ago, he developed *Staphylococcus aureus meningitis*, epidural abscess, and pneumonia. During his hospitalization, Bishop P developed quadriplegia, respiratory failure, renal failure, and persistent fevers. After he returned home, his wife worked part time while also providing home care. His daughter stopped her graduate studies to devote herself to his care.

Ten months later, Bishop P was admitted with urosepsis from *Enterobacter cloacae*. His course was complicated by hypotension, respiratory arrest, stroke, and seizures.

He was discharged, but returned to the hospital after three

weeks because of persistent fevers. During a five-week hospital stay, he developed ventilatory and renal failure, which required intubation and dialysis. Despite multiple courses of antibiotics, his blood cultures remained positive for *Enterobacter cloacae*, which are resistant to all antibiotics. His ascites fluid cultures also remained positive for several organisms. As a complication of his antibiotics, he developed autoimmune hemolytic anemia and thrombocytopenia, which required daily infusions of red cells and platelets. He also developed a total body rash, caused by a medication for his seizures. His skin sheared away around his bandages and electrocardiogram leads. The physicians predicted that he would not survive the hospitalization and that attempts at cardiopulmonary resuscitation (CPR) would be futile and disfigure his body.

Bishop P could not state his preferences for care. His family insisted that everything be done, because he believed that all life was sacred.

Bishop P's family wanted to act in accordance with his lifelong values. Such substituted judgments are a legitimate basis for decisions when patients lack decision-making capacity and have not given clear advance directives.[17] Physicians should respect religiously based decisions by patients, because deeply held religious beliefs reflect a person's core values and identity. Choices based on religion, therefore, may meet clinicians' practical adaptation of even the most stringent legal standards of evidence.[18] However, physicians need sufficient information about the patient's religious beliefs to make specific clinical decisions. Individuals may hold idiosyncratic beliefs, even if they belong to religions with extensive doctrines regarding medical care. For instance, some Jehovah's Witnesses will accept blood transfusions if a court orders the transfusions.[19] Furthermore, people who share general beliefs, such as the sacredness of life, may differ in their preferences regarding specific medical technologies.[20]

Physicians can disrespect patients' and families' religious beliefs in several ways. Some doctors discount such beliefs. All members of the medical team should acknowledge the possibility of discrimination on the basis of religion. Religions like Roman Catholicism and Judaism, which have established doctrines and academic traditions, may be more respected in hospitals because their history and scholarship are familiar to highly educated professionals. Fundamentalist sects may suffer because they tend to lack a substantial body of academic writing. Non-Western religions may be dismissed as unfamiliar or too removed from Western medicine to affect medical care.

Physicians also fail to show respect if they accept decisions based on religion, without trying to understand the patient's beliefs. Physicians can ask how religion shapes decisions without denigrating the patient's or family's faith. For example, a physician might say to Bishop P's daughter, "I know that religion plays an important part in your father's life. I'd like to understand it better. Please help me learn more." When a surrogate wants everything done, the physician must clarify what is meant by everything, whether or not that preference is based on religion.

THE ROLE OF THE FAMILY

CASE 2 CONTINUED

> In private, Bishop P's wife said that she thought aggressive treatment was no longer in her husband's best interests. However, she felt constrained by her daughter. Mrs. P noted that her husband would never want her to jeopardize her relationship with their children.

Legally and ethically, Bishop P's wife had authority to act as his surrogate. Some healthcare workers suggested that, because Mrs. P was concerned about criticism from her family, she was not acting in the best interests of her husband. These clinicians believed that Mrs. P's primary responsibility should be to her husband, not to her daughter.

Surrogates and patients live within a family and a community. Their connections to others have both ethical and practical significance. Proponents of an ethic of care have argued that more attention should be paid to how decisions affect various relationships and that families should have greater authority in healthcare decisions.[21] Relationships among family members will survive after the patient's death. These relationships deserve respect, and physicians should support surrogates who try to maintain family harmony. From a pragmatic point of view, family dynamics may be more important than legal distinctions. Many surrogates, like Mrs. P, are reluctant to contradict the views of close relatives and will not make a decision without the concurrence of the extended family. Similarly, in case 1, Mr. A's partner, his designated proxy, deferred to the medical expertise of Mr. A's brother, the critical care nurse, and made decisions jointly with the patient's brother and mother. Surrogates who feel caught between the patient and the family may suffer considerable stress. Physicians should acknowledge this stress and either respond to it directly or call on other resources such as social workers, chaplains, or ECs.

FUTILITY

When surrogates insist on interventions that physicians consider inappropriate, physicians may use the concept of futility to justify forgoing care without the surrogate's consent.[22] However, the doctrine of futility has been criticized as ambiguous,[23] potentially unfair,[24] overly broad in practice,[25] counterproductive,[26] and incapable of resolving many disputes.[27] Medical futility resolves disagreements by fiat rather than by negotiation.[28] In the context of an ongoing relationship, the use of futility to justify unilateral medical decisions fosters conflict.

Case 2 illustrates an additional important problem with futility. Futility would not resolve the question of how to manage Bishop P's overall care. CPR was futile, because it would not restore effective circulation if Bishop P developed progressive hypotension while on antibiotics, transfusions, and vasopressors.[29] However, transfusions, antibiotics, and ventilation were not strictly futile.[30] Although these interventions would not enable the patient to leave the hospital, they did keep Bishop P alive, a goal the family attributed to the patient. In pragmatic terms, writing a do-not-resuscitate (DNR) order over the objections of the family would not resolve difficult decisions regarding these other interventions. Indeed, invoking futility to justify a DNR order would likely heighten mistrust by the family of the medical staff and worsen surrogates' already strained relationship with the healthcare team. However, physicians and nurses who did not agree with the goal of prolonging life felt increasingly frustrated. Mechanical ventilation contributed to the same sense of frustration among Mr. A's healthcare team. It would not enable Mr. A to receive a liver transplant or allow him to leave the intensive care unit (ICU). However, it could prolong his life.

For the healthcare workers who disagreed with the goal of prolonging these patients' lives, rather than allowing them to die in comfort, the problem was not that life support was ineffective. The problem was that it succeeded all too well in prolonging life. Strictly futile treatments rarely contribute to the frustration of providing ongoing care. If interventions fail to achieve any clinical objective, they will not be continued day after day.

Professional caregivers can address their frustration at providing ongoing intensive care by borrowing from some recent developments in the futility debate. Several communities have crafted policies for local healthcare institutions that stress the importance of fair procedures in such disputes, before the choices of well-informed surrogates may be overridden.[31] These procedures emphasize careful communication with surrogates and suggest that clinicians and community members who are not involved with the care of the patient need to be involved in resolving disputes. At least one such policy recommends advising the surrogates that judicial recourse is an option for intractable conflicts.[32]

LIMITING INTERVENTIONS
THAT CAUSE SUFFERING

Although negotiation may resolve the vast majority of disputes, some prove intractable. Fair procedures alone cannot substitute for a substantive rule about when it is appropriate for professional integrity and the healthcare team's view of nonmaleficence to trump respect for autonomy. We suggest that one substantive rule is to deny surrogate requests for interventions that increase the pain and suffering of the patient, without proportional medical benefit.

In case 2, the family's requests for interventions that caused suffering troubled caregivers. When Bishop P's skin began shearing away, the healthcare team felt that attempts at CPR would cause disfiguration, without preventing death. The caregivers' reaction was more than frustration over providing interventions whose benefits were fleeting; meanwhile, the team members believed that they were actively increasing the patient's suffering. Many healthcare workers believe that it is unethical for them to provide interventions that cause suffering, with no proportionate benefit.[33] The ethical guideline of nonmaleficence here combines with professional integrity to allow healthcare workers to refrain from an intervention that causes significant suffering and, in case 2, would prolong the patient's life for no more than one hour. This rationale may justify overriding the family and withholding interventions; although it will do so only rarely.

Some surrogates state that the patient believes suffering serves a spiritual purpose. Spiritual aspects of dying are important to patients and have not been well appreciated by physicians.[34] However, caregivers should examine surrogates' claims about the redemptive nature of suffering. Many patients who believe their illness serves a spiritual purpose will accept medications for pain and decline burdensome interventions. Furthermore, patients may accept that the suffering caused by terminal illness serves some higher good, without agreeing to medical interventions that cause additional suffering but provide limited benefits.

The philosophical issue is how to define the patient's best interests. Physicians claim that it is not in the patient's interest to receive interventions that cause significant pain and postpone death for only a few days. The family may contend that the patient would accept such suffering. First, physicians should ascertain whether the family is presenting the patient's own view of his best interests, or drawing inferences from the patient's general values and religious beliefs. General goals of care do not accurately predict patient choices in specific clinical scenarios.[35] To clarify the patient's own view of his best interests, physicians should inquire about specific, informed statements by the patient that he/she would want painful interventions that provide limited benefits. Clear and explicit patient preferences are not required in most states as the basis for surrogate decision making. However, a high evidentiary standard to support treatment choices that inflict pain can be justified to protect patients from experiencing unnecessary distress as they die. Such a strict standard is justified because the risk of causing a patient to suffer outweighs the risk of failing to respect an autonomous, unconventional decision. We stress that the ethical difficulty here is that the surrogates are asking clinicians to take active steps to increase the suffering of an incompetent patient, for the sake of clinical outcomes that are not usually considered to justify such risks. This situation therefore differs from cases in which patients themselves refuse pain medication or tolerate painful side effects to seek personal fulfillment and advance their own healthcare values. When patients make such requests, physicians can talk with them in detail. Such discussions can clarify several important issues. Do they really understand the consequences of their request? Are there unaddressed psychosocial or clinical issues that, if attended to, would lead the patients to change their minds? Because such discussions are not possible with patients who lack decision-making capacity, physicians should be more circumspect when surrogates make such requests. In situations like case 2, professional integrity and nonmaleficence permit clinicians to honor their obligation to relieve suffering despite surrogates' insistence on painful interventions.

PRACTICAL SUGGESTIONS FOR WORKING WITH INSISTENT SURROGATES

In the ICU, surrogates ultimately agree with recommendations to limit life-sustaining treatment in almost all cases.[36] What can physicians do to make mutually acceptable decisions more likely?

GIVE SURROGATES TIME TO UNDERSTAND NEW CIRCUMSTANCES BEFORE REQUESTING A DECISION

Surrogates are frequently given bad news in the context of being asked to limit life-sustaining interventions. If possible, the surrogates should be given time to absorb the new information before making a decision. This recommendation underscores the fact that physicians should give surrogates the same information about prognosis and medical options that the patient, if competent, would receive.

HELP SURROGATES ACCEPT NEW DEVELOPMENTS AND EXPRESS THEIR CONCERNS

The passage of time alone will not persuade surrogates to limit interventions. Physicians should use time to address the barriers to agreement. First, physicians must elicit and respond to the concerns and views of the entire family. Physicians usually need to hold family meetings to explain the medical situation and their treatment recommendations and to respond to relatives' concerns. Open-ended questions help relatives articulate their concerns. For example: 'As you think about your partner's condition, what concerns you the most? What do you hope for?" Physicians can also shift the focus to making the patient's death meaningful. Doctors might say, "Your father is so seriously ill that we would not be surprised if he died in the hospital. What would be left undone if he were to die suddenly?" Social workers or chaplains can also help a family reach closure. Effective techniques for empathic and sensitive communication with families and patients have been described.[37] These communication skills are ethically justified because they enhance the ability of surrogates to make informed decisions. Surrogates' decisions are ethically flawed if surrogates have concerns or needs that are not articulated or addressed or if they do not appreciate the possibility of goals of care other than prolongation of life per se. Furthermore, persuasion and deliberation are ethically appropriate because they respect the surrogates as moral agents.

SET TIME LIMITS

If surrogates do not agree to forgo life-sustaining interventions, they may accept time limits on therapeutic trials of new or ongoing interventions.[38] Studies indicate that this time can be relatively short. Of the 9 percent of families who disagreed with recommendations to withhold or withdraw support in one study, 80 percent accepted the recommendation within two to three days.[39] In a later study, 90 percent of families accepted a recommendation to withhold or withdraw life support within less than five days.[40] Even given these relatively short periods of time, we recommend that the time for surrogates to adjust to a dramatically worse prognosis be proportionate to the time that has been devoted to aggressive care. For example, case 1 involved months of preparation for the expected liver transplantation. Allowing the family a week or two to adjust is a relatively small use of additional resources.

COMPROMISE ABOUT WITHDRAWING LIFE-SUSTAINING INTERVENTIONS

A common compromise involves not adding or increasing interventions but not withdrawing them.[41] Although law and ethics do not distinguish between withholding and withdrawing life support, the emotional difference may impress families. Willingness to continue interventions also may allay suspicions about physicians' motives for recommending limits to care. The rapid spread of managed care has raised public concern that physicians may be more concerned with saving money than benefiting the patient.[42]

REMAIN SENSITIVE TO ETHNIC AND CULTURAL ISSUES

Bishop P and his family were African Americans. Ethnic factors can be significant in end-of-life care. For example, African Americans and Hispanic Americans complete advance directives or wish to forgo life support less frequently than patients with other ethnic backgrounds.[43] Among African Americans, these differences may reflect mistrust caused by a history of discrimination and limited access to medical care.

Once ethnic or cultural issues have been identified, physicians should take practical steps to address them. Rather than leave concerns and suspicions unspoken, physicians might ask: "Many African Americans worry that they will not receive the care they need. How do you feel about that?" Physicians should not immediately try to reassure the family that all appropriate care will be provided. Instead, doctors may first need to listen and express empathy: "Is it distressing to think that you may not get the care you need?" Addressing issues of mistrust directly may demonstrate to family members that the doctor understands their concerns.

NEGOTIATE INTRACTABLE DISPUTES

Studies indicate that negotiation and compromise will resolve almost all disagreements between surrogates and physicians.[44] For this reason, the rare cases that cannot be resolved should not dictate the guidelines for approaching the majority of these disputes. The two cases we presented were considered intractable when they were first referred to the EC. Thus, the above suggestions may succeed in resolving even [apparently] intractable disagreements.

For cases that cannot be negotiated, three outcomes are possible. Either the physicians can compromise and continue to provide interventions; the family can compromise and agree to forgo some interventions; or one side can seek judicial involvement. We think that, in most cases, it will be more reasonable and appropriate for the physicians to compromise than for the surrogates to do so. The case for continuing life-prolonging interventions is strongest when the patient had previously given clear and specific directives that pertain to such a situation, when the surrogates believe that patient would not have changed his mind, and when the patient's preferences are founded on deeply held religious or personal moral beliefs. Judicial intervention is unlikely to resolve questions about care for moribund individuals in a timely manner, and courts are likely to look unfavorably on physicians and hospitals that seek injunctive relief to discontinue life-sustaining interventions.[45] Furthermore, going to court has its own side effects, because it places the family and healthcare workers in adversarial roles and delays the resolution of the case. However, as discussed, we believe one exception to the general guideline of physician compromise is that physicians should be able to refuse to increase the suffering of a moribund patient.

CONCLUSION

When surrogates for incompetent patients request interventions that physicians do not recommend, advance directives, legally appointed surrogates, or use of futility may offer little practical assistance. Physicians may be torn between their ethical obligation to respect delegated autonomy and their ethical obligation to maintain professional integrity by not harming their patients without corresponding benefit. Resolving this ethical dilemma requires negotiation with the community of surrogates, and thus this negotiation becomes an ethical obligation of its own. A negotiated understanding of the patient's best interests offers the best protection for the relationship between surrogates and physicians.

NOTES

1. See, for example, *In re Quinlan*, 335 A.2d 647 (N.J. 1976); *In re Conroy*, 486 A.2d 1209 (N.J. 1985); and *Cruzan v. Director, Missouri Department of Health*, 497 U.S. 261 (1990).

2. B. Lo, *Resolving Ethical Dilemmas: A Guide for Clinicians* (Baltimore: Williams & Wilkins, 1995), pp. 71–72; President's Commission for the Study of Ethical Problems in Medicine and Biomedical and Behavioral Research, *Deciding to Forgo Life-Sustaining Treatment: A Report on the Ethical, Medical, and Legal Issues in Treatment Decisions* (Washington, D.C.: U.S. Government Printing Office, 1983), pp. 80–82.

3. See President's Commission, *Deciding to Forgo Life-Sustaining Treatment*.

4. See R. Steinbrook et al., "Preferences of homosexual men with AIDS for life-sustaining treatment," *N Engl J Med* 314 (1986): 457–60.

5. D. Molloy et al., "Decision making in the incompetent elderly: 'The daughter from California syndrome,'" *J Amer Geriatr Soc* 39 (1991): 396–99.

6. S. H. Miles, "Informed demand for 'non-beneficial' medical treatment," *N Engl J Med* 325 (1991): 512–15; J. Paris, R. K. Crone, and F. Reardon, "Physicians' refusal of requested treatment: The case of Baby

L," *N Engl J Med* 322 (1990): 1012–14; J. Curtis et al., "The use of medical futility rationale in do-not-attempt-resuscitation orders," *JAMA* 273 (1995): 124–28; and T. J. Prendergast and J. M. Luce, "Increasing incidence of withholding and withdrawal of life support from the critically ill," *Amer J Resp Crit Care Med* 155 (1997): 15–20.

7. H. Brody, "Medical futility: A useful concept?" in M. B. Zucker and H. D. Zucker, ed., *Medical Futility and the Evaluation of Life-Sustaining Treatment* (Cambridge: Cambridge University Press, 1997), pp. 1–14.

8. Ibid.

9. E. Pellegrino and D. C. Thomasma, *The Virtues in Medical Practice* (New York: Oxford University Press, 1993), p. 131.

10. T. L. Beauchamp and J. F. Childress, *Principles of Biomedical Ethics*, 4th ed. (New York: Oxford University Press, 1994), p. 471.

11. F. G. Miller and H. Brody, "Professional integrity and physician-assisted death," *Hastings Center Report* 25, no. 3 (1995): 8–17.

12. N. N. Dubler, "Mediation and managed care," *J Amer Geriatr Soc* 46 (1998): 359–64.

13. A. Sehgal et al., "How strictly do dialysis patients want their advance directives followed?" *JAMA* 267 (1992): 59–63.

14. See Lo, *Resolving Ethical Dilemmas*, pp. 130–34.

15. See G. Rubenfeld and S. Crawford, "Withdrawing life support from mechanically ventilated recipients of bone marrow transplants: A case for evidence-based guidelines," *Ann Int Med* 125 (1996): 625–33.

16. G. S. Fischer et al., "Can goals of care be used to predict intervention preferences in an advance directive?" *Arch Int Med* 157 (1997): 810–807.

17. *In re Conroy*, 486 A.2d 1209 (N.J. 1985).

18. M. Tonelli, "Substituted judgment in medical practice: Evidentiary standards on a sliding scale," *J Law, Med & Ethics* 25 (1997): 22–29.

19. Lo, *Resolving Ethical Dilemmas*, pp. 91–92.

20. R. Dworkin, *Life's Dominion: An Argument about Abortion, Euthanasia, and Individual Freedom* (New York: Alfred A. Knopf, 1993), p. 328.

21. See N. Jecker, "The role of intimate others in medical decision making," *Gerontologist* 30 (1990): 65–71; J. Hardwig, "Treating the brain dead for the benefit of the family," *J Clin Ethics* 2 (1991): 53–56; and J. Hardwig, "What about the family?" *Hastings Center Report* 20, no. 2 (1990): 5–10.

22. L. J. Schneiderman, N. S. Jecker, and A. R. Jonsen, "Medical futility: Its meaning and ethical implications," *Ann Int Med* 112 (1990): 949–54; and R. D. Truog, A. S. Brett, and J. Frader, "The problem with futility," *N Engl J Med* 326 (1992): 1560–64.

23. Lo, *Resolving Ethical Dilemmas*, pp. 73–81.

24. A. Alpers and B. Lo, "When is CPR futile?" *JAMA* 273 (1995): 156–58; and L. J. Schneiderman, N. S. Jecker, and A. R. Jonsen, "Medical futility: Response to critiques," *Ann Int Med* 125 (1996): 669–74.

25. See Curtis et al., "The use of medical futility rationale," pp. 124–28.

26. J. M. Luce, "Making decisions about the forgoing of life-sustaining therapy," *Amer J Res Crit Care Med* 156 (1997): 1715–18.

27. A. Halevy, R. Neal, and B. Brody, "The low frequency of futility in an adult intensive care unit setting," *Arch Int Med* 156 (1996): 100–104.

28. T. J. Prendergast, "Resolving conflicts surrounding end-of-life care," *New Horizons* 5 (1997): 62–71.

29. See Lo, *Resolving Ethical Dilemmas*, pp. 158–61; and Emergency Cardiac Care Committee and Subcommittee, American Heart Association, "Guidelines for cardiopulmonary resuscitation and emergency cardiac care VIII: Ethical considerations in resuscitation," *JAMA* 268 (1992): 2282–88.

30. Lo, *Resolving Ethical Dilemmas*, p. 163.

31. A. Havley and B. A. Brody, "A multi-institution collaborative policy on medical futility," *JAMA* 276 (1996): 571–74; and D. J. Murphy and E. Barbour, "GUIDe (Guidelines for the Use of Intensive Care in Denver): A community effort to define futile and inappropriate care," *New Horizons* 2 (1994): 326–31.

32. See Bay Area Network of Ethics Committees (BANEC), "Conflict resolution guidelines from the nonbeneficial treatment working group," *West J Med* 170 (1999).

33. S. Braithwaite and D. Thomasma, "New guidelines on forgoing life-sustaining treatment in incompetent patients: An anti-cruelty policy," *Ann Int Med* 104 (1986): 711–15.

34. "Religious groups tackle end-of-life issues," *Last Acts: Care and Caring at the End of Life Quarterly Publication* (fall 1998): 1–2.

35. Fischer et al., "Can goals of care be used to predict intervention preferences in an advance directive?" pp. 801–807.

36. See Prendergast and Luce, "Increasing incidence of withholding

and withdrawing of life support," pp. 15–20; and N.G. Smedira et al., "Withholding and withdrawal of life support from the critically ill," *N Engl J Med* 322 (1990): 309–15.

37. P. M. Dunn and W. Levinson, "Discussing futility with patients and families," *J Gen Int Med* 11 (1996): 689–93.

38. Prendergast, "Resolving conflicts," pp. 62–71.

39. Smedira et al., "Withholding and withdrawal of life support," pp. 309–15.

40. Prendergast, "Resolving conflicts," pp. 62–71.

41. See D. A. Asch, J. Hansen-Flaschen, and R. N. Lanken, "Decisions to limit or not to continue life-sustaining treatment by critical care physicians in the United States: Conflicts between physicians' practices and patients' wishes," *Amer J Res Crit Care Med* 153 (1995): 288–92.

42. Prendergast, "Resolving conflicts," pp. 62–71.

43. R. V. Caralis et al., "The influence of ethnicity and race on attitudes toward advance directives, life-prolonging treatments, and euthanasia," *J Clin Ethics* 4 (1993): 155–65; L. J. Blackhall et al., "Ethnicity and attitudes toward patient autonomy," *JAMA* 274 (1995): 820–25; and S. M. Rubin et al., "Increasing completion of the durable power of attorney for health care: A randomized controlled trial," *JAMA* 271 (1994): 209–12.

44. Smedira et al., "Withholding and withdrawal of life support," pp. 309–15; and Prendergast, "Resolving conflicts," pp. 62–71.

45. G. J. Annas, "Asking the courts to set the standard of emergency care—The case of Baby K," *N Engl J Med* 330 (1994): 1542–45.

19

COMMENTARY
Anxieties as a Legal Impediment to the Doctor-Proxy Relationship

Marshall B. Kapp

Law-related anxieties among some physicians may affect how they behave toward patients and their proxies. Legal fears, whether based on an accurate understanding of applicable law or on misperceptions[1] about what the law really permits or requires, can influence the relationship between physicians and patients' proxies because these fears prompt physicians to give too much or too little deference to proxy decisions. Erring in either direction can contribute to adverse consequences for certain patients.

This commentary aims to outline some of the situations in which the physician-proxy relationship may be skewed negatively because of professional anxieties about legal entanglements. It then enumerates several strategies for addressing the problems of both undue and insufficient physician deference to proxy decision makers.

Reprinted from *Journal of Law, Medicine & Ethics* 27, no. 1 (spring 1999): 69–74, by permission of the American Society of Law, Medicine & Ethics. All rights reserved.

FAMILIES AS PLAINTIFFS

Physician anxiety about patients' family members as potential plaintiffs may be sharpest in cases of patients who are cognitively and/or emotionally incapacitated. These patients need a proxy to speak for them.[2] Especially for older patients in institutional settings, some physicians' legal risk aversion could bias them toward relying on proxies—particularly family members—to make decisions. Sometimes, this practice substitutes for a careful assessment of the patient's own functional capacity.[3]

If a question is raised about a patient's decisional capacity, some physicians may become fearful of potential liability for proceeding with medical interventions on the sole basis of the patient's own express wishes. In such circumstances, physicians could insist on immediate judicial appointment of a formal substitute decision maker, but this approach is contrary to the "least restrictive or intrusive alternative" position.[4]

In the decision-making process involving the critically ill and dying, patients' family members can disrupt the harmonious end-of-life care with demands for futile or otherwise unreasonable medical interventions. These demands may present questions about liability among medical professionals.[5] Suspicions about one's legal position can cloud the relationship between physicians and the families of critically ill and dying patients, and may manifest themselves in treatment options being provided in accordance with the family member whose preferences are the most aggressive—whether or not that person is an appointed healthcare agent or a legal surrogate. This bias is exemplified by one practitioner:

> I have in my practice an individual who has cost approximately $2.5 million to maintain over the past six years. During the time I have followed her, she has not moved, spoken, or given any indication of consciousness. She is being supported by a tube in

her windpipe attached to a respirator, by a tube in her stomach to continuously feed her, and by around-the-clock nursing care. This is not the wish of her providers, who have repeatedly requested that she be allowed to die. The family has insisted that all of this be done, *and in our present environment there is no good way to stop this futility.*[6]

In other words, adherence to the wishes of patients is perceived as a path by some physicians to avoid inquiries by risk managers or lawsuits by disgruntled family members.[7]

In end-of-life care, physicians can seek family consensus on treatment options even if there is a valid advance directive that states clearly a desire to forgo aggressive resuscitation measures. Such desires to avoid potential litigation prompted Christine K. Cassel to remark:

The problem often is that physicians hide behind their fear of malpractice any time an uncomfortable circumstance comes up. Doctors all make very bad lawyers, but that does not stop us from talking about it all the time. So doctors are always saying, "I do not want to be sued," and beads of sweat are quite common.[8]

At the other end of the spectrum, physicians can use legal apprehensions as a pretext for conduct that is driven wholly or partly by other forces, such as physicians' own psychological needs. In end-of-life decision making, deviation from patients' wishes may be blamed on legal concerns, even though they really stem more from communication difficulties, an ongoing ambivalence about power and control in the physician-patient or physician-proxy relationship, and an attempt to define medical success in terms of survival rather than meaningfulness to the patient.[9]

LEGAL SOURCES OF LIABILITY

Perceptions that physicians should appease families' demands has been reinforced by several recent legal developments, which include court decisions in futility cases[10] and liability concerns related to discrimination under the Americans with Disabilities Act (ADA).[11]

Among futility cases,[12] *In the Matter of Baby K* has received the most attention. This case involved an anencephalic infant from whom physicians wanted to withhold resuscitation attempts in the event of cardiac arrest, because they felt that cardiopulmonary resuscitation would provide no benefit. Baby K's mother insisted that resuscitation be initiated if and when her daughter was brought to the hospital's emergency department. In a decision that has drawn pointed legal derision,[13] the court upheld the mother's right to insist that everything be done to keep her daughter alive.[14] Some physicians would interpret this decision expansively, arguing that it compels as much medical intervention as may be demanded. In fact, one physician wrote: "Unless there is some legal relief from this condition, most physicians will probably continue to 'do everything' if the family so instructs . . . whether or not they feel it is in the patient's best interest."[15]

The ADA introduced another unpredictable legal variable into the equation. It raises apprehension that the failure to provide aggressively the whole range of life-sustaining medical interventions for every patient could expose the physician to damages, on the grounds of unlawful discrimination in the provision of services. Speculation on this possibility and on related issues has also begun to appear in the professional literature.[16] One commentator has reasoned that, given the expansive protective shadow cast by the ADA, "[T]he physician's standing may not be equal in stature to that of the family and would not justify unilateral cessation of treatment without a court order."[17]

Regulations implementing the ADA authorize disabled

patients to decline services that would otherwise be mandated by the ADA, but expressly refuse to authorize disabled persons' guardians or representatives to decline medical treatment on a disabled person's behalf.[18] The law also makes clear that families cannot be punished for violation of the ADA, but that physicians and healthcare institutions can be held liable and sanctioned for regulatory transgressions.[19]

PROXIES AS A SOURCE OF LIABILITY

Deference to proxies' wishes resulting in undertreatment rather than overtreatment of a patient is illustrated in one case involving a California nursing home.[20] Mrs. S was an eighty-five-year-old nursing home resident with Alzheimer's disease, arthritis, and hypothyroidism. Despite her conditions, she was socially active and functioned for the most part independently. Mrs. S was able to walk without help, needed minimal assistance with personal grooming, was continent, could carry on a conversation, and was generally alert but confused at times.

One day, Mrs. S's condition changed suddenly. She developed severe symptoms that led to a diagnosis after five days of an abscessed tooth. Mrs. S's adult son, who lived in a nearby suburb, was her naturally occurring surrogate. He refused to permit treatment (including transfer to a hospital), saying that he wanted no "heroic" intervention because his mother was just "existing." Neither the nursing home's director of nursing nor its medical director, both of whom were well aware of this situation as it unfolded, advocated for Mrs. S in the face of her son's refusal to approve care for the treatable but life-threatening infection. Instead, they acceded to the son's decision, and Mrs. S died a medically unnecessary, premature, painful death. The healthcare professionals justified their conduct on the grounds that, had they disregarded the son's wishes, he might have sued them.

Two somewhat similar instances of deference to proxies have been described by clinical ethicist Kenneth Simpson.[21] He describes a sixty-one-year-old woman who was unconscious and ventilator-dependent after a cardiac arrest. One week later, the family requested termination of life support. The medical team acquiesced, even though it had insufficient time to determine properly the patient's prognosis. Fortunately, an improvement in the patient's mental status was observed shortly before the ventilator was to be disconnected. She was weaned from it and regained the ability to communicate and follow commands.

In the second case, Simpson describes a family's demands to terminate mechanical ventilation for a patient dying of pneumonia related to acquired immune deficiency syndrome. The request would have superseded the patient's own wishes. The patient retained decisional capacity, but was too heavily sedated to participate in decisions. When sedatives were discontinued, the competent patient angrily rejected his family's request to withdraw the ventilator, and he remained capable of interaction for more than a week.

PHYSICIAN ACTIONS AS A SOURCE OF LIABILITY

In each of the situations, physicians relied on their understanding of the pertinent state healthcare agent/surrogate statute and judicial decisions interpreting that statute. When proxies are perceived as potential plaintiffs by physicians who know that the patient, because of medical condition, will not be able to assert his/her own rights, the proxies' wishes can assume preeminence for the wrong reasons. In such cases, the proxies are only accountable to themselves.

The foregoing discussion describes one side of the coin. However, the reverse can also be argued: proxies are not always obeyed by physicians.

Attorney Gere Fulton[22] describes a case in which proxy decisions arguably were given insufficient deference because of the physicians' legal anxieties. In *In re Gary Kramp*, Fulton explains, the attending physicians gave the patient's family (the naturally occurring surrogates)—who wanted life-sustaining medical intervention withdrawn from their dying relative—a hard time following hospital counsel's advice. That advice was based on a narrow interpretation of a state advance directive statute that was read to require that a patient be in a permanent vegetative state for at least a year before treatment could be legally abated. This case exemplifies the difficulties that may occur because of legislation,[23] as exacerbated by risk managers who discourage following the wishes of well-intentioned proxies.

In one of several conversations with the hospital's attorney, Fulton (negotiating on the family's behalf) was told: "[W]e're getting a heinous result, but we're doing the right [risk management] thing."[24] After a court ordered the physicians and hospital to comply with the proxies' request to refuse treatment,[25] Fulton concluded: "This is a tragic waste of time, energy, and money for all who are consigned to dwell in this legal wonderland."[26]

STRATEGIES

Physicians legitimately want reasonable legal certainty when making life-and-death decisions. These are questions about such matters as who has the legal authority (1) to make valid healthcare decisions permitting or refusing specific interventions; (2) to receive medical information about the patient; (3) to claim or waive the right of confidentiality regarding the patient's medical information; and (4) to accept responsibility for paying the bill for services provided.

The legal risks entailed in treating patients absent clarity on these points about decisional authority may be exaggerated by some, because treatment often occurs within legal "gray zones." According to calculations by Alan Meisel, between 0.2 and 0.5 percent of all American patient deaths since 1976 have been litigated in any manner, and between thirty-seven and fifty-five in ten million have been litigated to the point of yielding an appellate decision.[27] These statistics notwithstanding, a desire for prospective certainty concerning rights and obligations on the part of physicians is understandable.

To the extent that anxiety about legal liability impairs the doctor-proxy relationship, strategies to address those apprehensions need to be identified. These strategic approaches can be regulatory, educational, or administrative, and are not mutually exclusive.

The regulatory approach would attempt to address law-related problems by enacting more law. Under the theory that any shortcomings in the doctor-proxy relationship are at least partially attributable to bad public policy decisions reflected in present statutes and regulations, or to inartful drafting of the law, we can write better laws to cure those shortcomings. There is little evidence of success in other attempts at legal reform;[28] moreover, some difficulties in the doctor-proxy relationship may lie less in the failings of the applicable law than in how physicians, administrators, and risk managers misinterpret the applicable law. Finally, reliance on a regulatory solution could further confuse rather than improve the existing situation.

If misunderstanding of the actual statutes impedes proper doctor-proxy interaction, educational efforts targeted at physicians and proxies about their rights and responsibilities may be productive. Institutional and agency attorneys and risk managers, on whose advice physician behavior is sometimes predicated, should also be targeted. Information dissemination could convey, in understandable terms, a realistic perspective about actual and perceived legal risks to the involved participants. Initiating educational efforts preemptively, which is desirable, will face tough sailing but should be pursued.

Administrative approaches to improve the doctor-proxy relationship could include developing, disseminating, and enforcing institutional, agency, and office policies and procedures pertaining to various facets of the relationship. The developmental phase of these policies and procedures would provide a valuable educational exercise for the drafters. Protocol content would provide prospective and concurrent guidance, and a source of support, for the ethically and legally proper handling of specific, potentially contentious issues as they emerge during patient care. Besides contributing to good ethical processes and results, this approach could have tangible risk management benefits by providing evidence of good faith conduct in the event that the propriety of a physician's interaction with a proxy were later challenged.

Administrative policies and procedures by themselves may not be enough to counter some physicians' belief that "we're the deep pockets, so we're the ones who will be sued." Institutional practice, in the form of positive administrative role modeling, may convince physicians of sufficient support and risk sharing to take actions that some of them would consider ethically correct but legally courageous.

Finally, we need a research agenda to examine the impact of legal anxieties on the functioning of the doctor-proxy relationship. We should explore empirically such questions as how physicians derive their ideas about the law, the extent to which these perceptions are accurate, how these perceptions really affect physician interaction with proxies and care for patients, and the effects (intended and unintended) of particular policy and practice interventions of the sort enumerated above. Attorneys and professional health services researchers with qualitative and quantitative expertise ought to work together—employing the analytical tools of therapeutic jurisprudence[29]—to analyze data on these questions so to inform policymakers,[30] educators, administrators, risk managers, and physicians.

NOTES

1. Regarding physicians' misperceptions about legal standards of care, see, for example, B. A. Liang, "Assessing medical malpractice jury verdicts: A case study of an anesthesiology department," *Cornell Journal of Law and Public Policy* 7 (1997): 121–64.

2. See, for example, L. J. Schneiderman and H. Teetzel, "Who decides who decides? When disagreement occurs between the physician and the patient's appointed proxy about the patient's decision-making capacity," *Arch Int Med* 155 (1995): 793–96; and L. C. Hanson et al., "Impact of patient incompetence on decisions to use of withhold life-sustaining treatment," *Amer J Med* 97 (1994): 23S–41.

3. See M. B. Kapp, "Liability issues and assessment of decision-making capability in nursing home patients," *Amer J Med* 89 (1990): 639–42.

4. See W. C. Schmidt Jr., *Guardianship: The Court of Last Resort for the Elderly and Disabled* (Durham: Carolina Academic Press, 1995); and G. J. Annas and J. Densberger, "Competence to refuse medical treatment: Autonomy versus paternalism," *University of Toledo Law Review* 15 (1984): 561–96.

5. See, for example, D. W. Molloy et al., "Decision making in the incompetent elderly: The daughter from California syndrome," *J Amer Geriatr Soc* 39 (1991): 396–99.

6. B. Fowkes, Letter, "The right to die," *Newsweek*, September 19, 1994, p. 16 (emphasis added).

7. See D. T. Watts, "The family's will or the living will: Patient self-determination in doubt," *J Amer Geriatr Soc* 40 (1992): 533–34; and J. Ely et al., "The physician's decisions to use tube feedings: The role of the family, the living will, and the Cruzan decision," *J Amer Geriatr Soc* 40 (1992): 471–75.

8. End of Life Issues and Implementation of Advance Directives Under Health Care Reform: Hearings Before the Senate Comm. on Finance, 103d Cong. 43 (1994) (testimony of Christine K. Cassel, M.D., Chair, Department of Geriatrics, Mount Sinai School of Medicine).

9. See T. Gilligan and T.A. Raffin, "Whose death is it, anyway?" *Ann Int Med* 126 (1996): 137–41.

10. See, for example, J. F. Daar, "Medical futility and implications for physician autonomy," *Amer J Law & Med* 21 (1995): 221–40.

11. Americans with Disabilities Act, 42 U.S.C. SS 1210112213 (1990).

12. For example, *In re Wanglie*, No. PX-283 (Minn. Dist. Ct. 1991); *In re Jane Doe*, 418 S.E.2d 3 (Ga. 1992); *In re Doe*, C.A. No. D-93064 (Ga. Super. Ct. 1991); and *Duensing* v. *Southwest Texas Medical Hospital*, No. SA-CA-1 119 (W.D. Tex. 1988). See also A. M. Capron, "Baby Ryan and virtual futility," *Hastings Center Report* 25, no. 2 (1995): 20–21.

13. See, for example, G. J. Annas, "Asking the courts to set the standard of emergency care—The case of Baby K," *N Engl J Med* 330 (1994): 1542–45.

14. *In the Matter of Baby K*, 16 F.3d 590 (4th Cir. 1994).

15. R. A. Fronduti, Letter, "Do everything," *Ann Int Med* 121 (1994), p. 900.

16. See, for example, D. Orentlicher, "Destructuring disability: rationing of health care and unfair discrimination against the sick," *Harvard Civil Rights–Civil Liberties Law Review* 31 (1996): 49–87.

17. P. G. Peters Jr., "When physicians balk at futile care: Implications of the disability rights law," *Northwestern University Law Review* 91 (1997): 841.

18. 28 C.F.R. S 35.130(e) (1999).

19. Ibid.

20. J. Kayser-Jones and M. B. Kapp, "Advocacy for the mentally impaired elderly: A case study analysis," *Amer J Law & Med* 14 (1989): 353–76.

21. See K. Simpson, "Health care surrogate laws," *N Engl J Med* 328 (1993): 1200.

22. See G. B. Fulton, "The non-declarant in a PVS: Adventures in Ohio's legal wonderland," *Ohio Northern Law Review* 20 (1994): 571–95.

23. See M. B. Kapp, "State statutes limiting advance directives: Death warrants or life sentences?" *J Amer Geriatr Soc* 40 (1992): 722–26.

24. Fulton, "The non-declarant in a PVS," p. 581.

25. Compare this approach with that exhibited by the Supreme Court of Wisconsin. See *In the Matter of Edna M.F.* v. *Eisenberg*, 210 Wis. 2d 557, 563 N.W.2d 485 (1997), holding that, if an incompetent patient is not in a persistent vegetative state, maximally aggressive medical interventions may not be discontinued in the absence of an advance directive or other specific prior statement of the patient's wishes under the precise circumstances.

26. Fulton "The non-declarant in a PVS," p. 595. A description of this

sort of problem has also been presented from the perspective of a patient's daughter. See E. Hansot, "A letter from a patient's daughter," *Ann Int Med* 125 (1996): 149–51.

27. A. Meisel, "The 'right to die': A case study in American law-making," *European Journal of Health Law* 3 (1996): 68–69.

28. But see D. P. Kessler and M. B. McClellan, "The efects of malpractice pressure and liability reforms on physicians' perceptions of medical care," *Law and Contemporary Problems* 60 (1997): 105 (emphasis added), claiming "that law reforms affect physicians' *attitudes*, both by reducing the probability of an encounter with the liability system, and by changing the nature of the experience of being sued for those physicians who defend against malpractice claims."

29. See generally D. B. Wexler and B. J. Winick, eds., *Law in a Therapeutic Key: Developments in Therapeutic Jurisprudence* (Durham: Carolina Academic Press, 1996).

30. Compare Symposium, "Lies, damn lies and statistics: How empirical research shapes health law and policy," *Indiana Law Review* 31(1998): 9–142.

2 0

COMMENTARY
From Contract to Covenant in Advance-Care Planning

Joseph J. Fins

Now here's a good way to do concrete ethics: Don't just tell stories interpreted in the old words of ethical theories. Show the intimate feelings of the storyteller, *me*.[1]

As a physician who cares for patients and families at the end of life, I have realized that the ethical theories describing the patient-proxy relationship can fail to give adequate guidance to patients or their potential proxies.[2] Often couched in a legalistic or *contractual* framework, the prevailing theory can be difficult to translate into clinical practice and is sometimes inaccessible to patients, proxies, and their physicians. In this commentary, I suggest a *covenantal* view of the patient-proxy relationship to complement the prevailing conception of this relationship.[3] My intention is to improve the quality of advance care planning by offering patients and their proxies a framework that reflects other important relationships in their lives.

Reprinted from *Journal of Law, Medicine & Ethics* 27, no. 1 (spring 1999): 46–51, by permission of the American Society of Law, Medicine & Ethics. © 1999. All rights reserved.

FIDELITY, WISDOM, AND LOVE

When I imagine when I might need to rely on my healthcare proxy, I hope that she will step forward and represent my interests with fidelity, wisdom, and love. I hope she takes account of my wishes, our life together, and the medical facts that have been shared with her. I do not want her to be forced to adhere slavishly to what I might have said or written.

As I imagine her deliberations, I do not expect them to be an exercise in rationality, informed by prevailing ethical theory. I suspect theory will be nearly irrelevant to her. Indeed, if a medical ethicist came to the bedside and counseled her to make decisions based on the prevailing standards for surrogate decision making, I can imagine her asking him why he had stopped by. She would be helped less by concepts like expressed wishes, substituted judgment, and best interests than by recalling our intertwined lives and the challenges that we had faced together. Instead of trying to reconstruct what I would do if I were still capable of making decisions, she would take a broader view of her newfound responsibility. In her deliberations, she would be guided by an intimate knowledge of who I was and the values that had informed my life's work and conduct. All of this would be more important to her than a cryptic comment about ventilators or feeding tubes.

Because she alone would have knowledge of our shared life, I would resent any theoretical formulation that would constrain her ability to make choices on my behalf. Such intrusions would violate our privacy and trump the bond that established our relationship.

In sketching out these hopes for my proxy, I have deviated from conventional norms. These conventional norms, which might loosely be termed the *contractual* model of the patient-proxy relationship, favor the promotion of patient self-determination through the agency of the patient's proxy.[4] This framework favors the patient's expressed wishes or the invocation of substituted judgment, with a best-interests standard directing care when patient preferences are scant or unknown. These standards leave little room for creativity. The proxy is not seen as a patient intimate but rather as a sterile instrument who accurately conveys patient preferences.

This contractual view is most appropriate when the patient's preferences are clear or when a patient has not appointed a surrogate who knows him well. In the first case, a rigid decision-making hierarchy prevents the proxy from deviating too far from the patient's preferences. In the second, contractual constraints on decision making serve to protect the patient from the uninformed, ill-chosen, or even mischievous proxy.

In this way, the contractual framework *appropriately* protects the vulnerable patient from outright violations of his preferences. It is not, however, the ideal way to conceptualize the proxy's obligations when the situation is morally ambiguous and the proxy believes that strict adherence to the patient's express preferences violates the patient's intentions and the proxy's obligations.

In these difficult situations, the constraints placed on the proxy may deprive the patient of the fullest judgment of the person best suited to represent him. Although we need a mechanism for proxy decision making when the patient does not have an intimate as a proxy, why should we limit ourselves to a minimalist view of the proxy's responsibilities when that relationship needs to become much more? The need to protect a vulnerable incapacitated patient should not deprive others of an opportunity for the fullest expression of the patient's trust in his proxy.

In my clinical experience, not all proxy designations are the same and the contractual model does not accommodate the full range of relationships that can lead to a proxy designation. We need a complementary conceptualization that addresses the experiences of an informed and loving proxy confronted with a difficult moral choice. Viewing the patient-proxy relationship as a contractual arrangement that has the potential to become what I consider a covenantal relationship can provide this perspective.

I offer this covenantal perspective as an aspirational model to complement the prevailing contractual model that dominates current thinking about advance directives. I endorse the centrality of patient self-determination in advance care planning and caution against the unjustified trumping of patient preferences.[5] Nonetheless, many cases of surrogate decision making present unclear choices that require the proxy's judgment and discretion. These complex cases will not be resolved through the deductive application of abstract ethical principles, like autonomy or beneficence, but from a more inductive and *clinically pragmatic* process of moral problem solving that instructs us to examine the facts and circumstances of particular cases to reach ethically appropriate decisions.[6]

We can better prepare proxies for these unanticipated challenges if we introduce a covenantal perspective into advance care planning. My objective is not to make all proxy designations covenantal, but to make each of these choices more reflective of the life narratives that inform the patient's choice of a proxy.

CONTRACTS AND COVENANTS

Viewing the patient-proxy relationship as potentially both contractual and covenantal requires an appreciation of the often subtle difference between a contract and a covenant. At times, this difference seems semantic, as in the terms *marriage contract* and *marriage covenant.*

The primary definitions of contract and covenant in the *Oxford English Dictionary* suggest that the terms are synonyms. *Contract* is defined as "a binding agreement between two or more parties; . . . A document in which an agreement is set out for signature by the parties concerned." A *covenant* is similarly described as "a mutual agreement between two or more persons to do or refrain from doing certain acts; the undertaking of either party in such an agreement."[7]

If we move beyond these principle definitions, we can appreciate that, even though contracts and covenants have common elements, each emphasizes different aspects of complex relationships. Philip Hallie distinguishes the contractual from the covenantal in *Tales of Good and Evil, Help and Harm*. There, he addresses this distinction as it relates to relationships between those who provide help and those who need it.[8]

Drawing on his earlier work,[9] Hallie considers the difference between contractual and covenantal help. Contractual help, according to him, has an economic or legal component. It is not purely voluntary; rather, it is sustained by a *quid pro quo* such as a payment or a legal constraint. Covenantal help, in contrast, is freely given and is what he calls "gratuitous helping."

Echoing this sentiment, William F. May suggests that a contract is less morally compelling than a covenant.[10] May observes that

> as opposed to the instrument of contract that presupposes agreement reached on the basis of self-interest, covenantal ethics may require one to be available to the covenant partner above and beyond the measure of self-interest; thus covenantal ethics has an element of the gratuitous in it.[11]

Using the physician's professional relationship and obligations to individuals and society at large as an example, May considers the benefits of a contractualistic and a covenantal ethic.[12] He explains that contractual relationships are easier to regulate and tend to be less hierarchical than ones based on blind trust or faith. They promote informed consent and establish a greater degree of symmetry against unequal powers. This is often accomplished through the exchange of expertise for payment.

Writing about the doctor-patient relationship, May hopes that the physician's role rises to the level of a covenant to overcome "self-interested minimalism" that only functions when matched with a *quid pro quo*. He argues that a covenantal approach is the only way to address unexpected contingencies, which may not be explicitly delineated in a contract.

COVENANTS AND FAITHFUL RELATIONSHIPS

A covenantal approach can be helpful in relationships predicated on trust. Unlike a legal contract, explicitly spelling out obligations between parties to avoid uncertainty or possible distrust, a covenant presupposes faithfulness. Such faithfulness can be understood in either a religious or secular context. According to the *Baker Encyclopedia of the Bible*, *covenant* is defined as an "arrangement between two parties involving mutual obligations; especially the arrangement that established the relationship between God and His people expressed in grace first with Israel and then with the church."[13]

In this manner, a covenantal relationship is similar to the relationships that exist within families. In family life, one's roles and obligations are dictated by birth and motivated by mutually reciprocating responsibilities. A mother who cares for a sick child or the adult child who attends to her widowed mother may do so out of love and filial duty. Each act of devotion is part of a set of obligations binding one generation to the next. These responsibilities are not agreed to in advance. They are instead a birthright, inherited much like the biblical covenant between God and His people.

This abiding devotion is characteristic of covenantal relationships. Unlike a contract, which may be conditional and time limited, a covenant between individuals is based on "faithfulness" that cannot easily be severed:

> The essence of covenant is to be found in a particular kind of relationship between persons. Mutual obligations characterize that kind of relationship. Thus a covenant relationship is not merely a mutual acquaintance but a commitment to responsibility and action. A key word in Scripture to describe that commitment is "faithfulness," acted out in a context of abiding friendship.[14]

With this definition of covenant, we can return to the distinction between a marriage contract and marriage covenant and agree with Hegel that a marriage that remains a contract is not a marriage. Hegel maintained that to subsume marriage under the concept of contract was "shameful." He argued that

> marriage, so far as its essential basis is concerned, is not a contractual relation. On the contrary, though marriage begins in contract, it is precisely a contract to transcend the standpoint of contract, the standpoint from which persons are regarded in their individuality as self-subsistent units.[15]

By this, Hegel implies that, although a contract formalizes or enables marriage vows, a marriage must become covenantal to fulfill truly those abiding vows.[16]

The same might be said of the covenantal relationship that can exist between the patient and proxy. Although it begins as a contractual relationship, the contract can evolve into a covenant when the patient and proxy understand the designation as an enduring and unifying set of obligations.[17]

When these reciprocal obligations are applied to the patient-proxy relationship, we can overcome the deminimist notion of a contract. The patient can expect that his proxy will "take [him] through to [his] death."[18] This is not a time-limited responsibility, but a set of mutual obligations. The patient is obliged to select an appropriate proxy and prepare her for the morally weighty role she will assume. The proxy, in turn, is obliged to fulfill her responsibilities to the dependent patient.

When capacity is lost, the covenant between patient and proxy is embodied in shared memory. Memories remain an enduring legacy to the proxy who must draw on this inheritance for guidance.

Viewed covenantally, this is a forceful mandate for planning and prevention and for choosing one's proxy well.[19] It counters the trivialization of the proxy designation that can occur and requires that the patient minimize the burden imposed on the proxy. It also is a mandate for the clinician to assist the patient and proxy with this process.[20]

It is remarkable to observe that some patients neglect to inform their proxies that they have been chosen or fail to speak with them in more than a cursory manner about the moral responsibility that they have given them. These lapses can impose an untenable burden on the unlucky and unprepared proxy; and they breach the covenant that should ideally bind the patient and proxy.

SOURCES OF MORAL AUTHORITY IN THE PATIENT-PROXY RELATIONSHIP

We usually understand advance directives and the proxy's role in particular through external contractual constraints.[21] But, in complex cases, a proxy's legal authority to act may remain morally ambiguous. In such cases, a proxy will have unimpeachable legal and contractual authority, but remain uncertain about how best to fulfill the obligations. When this occurs, it is helpful to transcend the contractual and to act covenantally.[22] A covenant can provide moral guidance because although:

> Contracts are external; covenants are internal to the parties involved. We sign contracts to discharge them expediently. Covenants cut deeper into personal identity.[23]

The place of covenantal thinking becomes apparent if we consider the case of an octogenarian with mild to moderate Alzheimer's disease. The patient completed an advance directive five years before becoming demented. She was admitted to a hospital after fracturing her hip. Her husband, who is her healthcare agent, consents to surgery. Her intraoperative course is unremarkable, and the procedure is successful. However, postoperatively, she does not wake up in the recovery room.

Once awake, it is apparent that she has become encephalopathic with a profoundly impaired mental status. Her physicians perform a diagnostic work-up and find no clear etiology for her change in mental status. They speculate that she might have sustained a fat embolism to the brain during the surgery.

After a couple of weeks of no meaningful change in her mental status, the patient's husband fears the worst. He asks that her artificial nutrition and hydration be withdrawn. But, as this request is made, the patient slowly begins to come out of her stupor. Her physicians are reluctant to remove nutritional support because they believe that she may be recovering her mental status. Concerned that her recovery would be retarded by the withdrawal of food and water, they meet with the proxy, intending to counter his request. They also request the assistance of the institution's ethics committee (EC).

In the meeting with the proxy and his family, the physicians learn that the patient did not want to be placed on artificial nutrition and hydration. This wish was substantiated by the standard advance directive, which contained the following statements under an "optional instructions" section:

> I do not want mechanical ventilation.
> I do not want cardiopulmonary resuscitation.
> I do not want artificial nutrition and hydration.

Based on this evidence, the physicians assembled at the scheduled meeting of the EC have a change of heart. They now believe that the withdrawal of artificial nutrition and hydration is ethically justified.

The EC agrees that the proxy has the legal right to make this decision, but it suggests how the proxy could use his authority more productively. The EC wants him to consider as fully as possible the implications of any decision he might make. In its deliberations, the EC maintains that the proxy can fulfill his obligations by (1) continuing treatment in the hopes of a recovery; (2) seeking to minimize pain and suffering; or (3) following the patient's previously expressed wishes to be protected from disproportionately burdensome interventions. Each choice is ethically acceptable as long as it is motivated by covenantal or "gratuitous helping" that achieved a patient-centered good.

To make a truly informed decision, the EC felt that the proxy would need to reflect on whether the patient had thought about forgoing artificial nutrition and hydration in her current state or if she were imminently dying. Artificial nutrition and hydration would merely prolong the dying process if she were critically ill; but, in this case, withholding artificial nutrition and hydration could impose a greater burden. It could lead to a catabolic state with its attendant risks of bedsores and poor wound healing.

The EC contended that a purely contractual view of the advance directive might not fully address the patient's situation. It appreciated that a strict reading might not have reflected the patient's true wishes and that to honor the patient's intent, physicians would need to turn to the proxy for guidance. The EC felt that the written instructions to forgo artificial nutrition and hydration needed to be *interpreted* by the proxy. With this in mind, it suggested that the patient's physicians inform the proxy of the consequences of the care options so that he could make a truly informed decision.

It made this recommendation recognizing that the proxy could contravene the patient's literal wishes. This risk was accepted because the EC viewed the patient's written directive as only a part of her advance care planning legacy. Given the circumstances, this *substantive* legacy had to be balanced against the *procedural* authority that came from having been designated her proxy.

To acknowledge the substance of her advance directive at the expense of the proxy's designation would discount an important dimension of the patient's advance care planning. It would foreclose the involvement of her proxy and turn her advance directive into a living will, with its near exclusive emphasis on literal instructions.

In this case, the patient's proxy was fortunate. Despite the tragedy that had befallen his beloved wife, he knew what she would have wanted. Once informed of the likely consequences of the care options, he instructed the physicians to withhold artificial nutrition and hydration. Though tragic, this case did not present the proxy with a difficult moral conflict, because the substantive and procedural sources of his moral authority as proxy were mutually reinforcing.

Sometimes, however, the proxy's procedural authority can appropriately trump the patient's articulated preferences. When this occurs, the covenant can legitimately take precedence over the contractual dimensions of advance care planning. This occurs in practice when physicians seek a proxy's interpretation even when a living will exists.

Consider the case of a sixty-year-old admitted to a hospital on a hot summer day with palpitations and a new right bundle branch block on his electrocardiogram (EKG). He has mild hypertension, for which he takes a diuretic, but is otherwise healthy. On admission to the cardiac unit, anxious and waiting for his family, he consents to a do-not-resuscitate (DNR) order. The patient's evaluation reveals that his potassium level is dangerously low and that this easily reversible electrolyte disturbance precipitated the EKG changes. Treatment is begun with intravenous potassium supplements and his cardiogram normalizes.

The patient's son, who is his proxy, later learns of the DNR designation. As a third-year medical student, he knows that although resuscitation is rarely successful, it would be most effective in this clinical circumstance. He asks his father to rescind the DNR order and explains his rationale. On hearing his son's explanation, the patient agrees to the change in his resuscitation status.

Once this is done, the son also tells his father that, had he gone into cardiac arrest, he would *not* have honored his decision to forgo resuscitation. To him, it seemed illogical that his father would want to avoid a potentially successful resuscitation. He suspected that, when his father consented to the DNR order, he was intending to avoid a lingering death or a persistent vegetative state. He did not believe that his father's decision had been truly informed.

He told his father that he felt morally obliged to act against his explicit wishes. He felt that his intercession would have been ethically appropriate given his superior knowledge of the medical facts. Indeed, for him, failure to do so would have been a violation of the trust his father had placed in him[24] and of the high value their family had always placed on independent thinking and reasoned exchange. True to form, when the father heard his son's perspective, he agreed.

Although anecdotal, the father's trust in his son's judgment points to an emerging empirical literature about how patients conceptualize their relationship with their proxies. According to Peter A. Singer et al.'s recent study of perceptions of advance care planning, patients tend to place their faith in those who will come to represent them.[25] They are not as wedded to notions of autonomy or the exercise of control. Instead, they want to relieve the burdens placed on others and reject traditional academic assumptions about how to approach advance care planning. This provocative work implicitly suggests that patients view the relationship with their proxies as a covenant and want their designated surrogates to transcend the contract when necessary.

Singer et al.'s findings also provide important insight into the SUPPORT study, which demonstrated the inability of advance directives to influence end-of-life practice patterns.[26] This often-cited study used the passage of the Patient Self-Determination Act of 1990, documentation, and nurse facilitators as *external* prompts to promote advance directives. Its focus, in my view, was almost exclusively on the contractual dimensions of advance care planning. These contractual interventions did not improve care or increase the use or influence of advance directives. But any conclusion about advance care planning that focuses on the contractual, at the expense of the covenantal, provides a mistaken assessment of how patients and proxies negotiate the actual challenges of advance care planning.

It is notable that SUPPORT investigators failed to highlight a subset of patients in their study for whom advance directives did seem to make a difference.[27] They observed that patients in their control group, who had advance directives prior to study enroll-ment, exhibited a heightened use of earlier DNR orders and a greater preference for palliative care.[28] These advance directives were not the by-product of an external experimental prompt, but were *naturally occurring* and emblematic of prospective decisions. They grew organically from preexisting relationships. It can be inferred that this effective subset of advance directives was more fully informed by internally motivated covenants than those that require a contractual or external prompt.

A more recent study confirms how advance directives influ-ence end-of-life practice patterns. This study found that patients with naturally occurring advance directives had statistically sig-nificant increases in DNR orders and the use of "comfort care plans."[29] These findings demonstrate the potential of prehospital advance care planning to enhance hospital decision making and end-of-life care. It also underscores the centrality of covenantal relationships to the success of advance directives.

CONCLUSION

The advantages of a covenantal approach highlight the problems with our current approach to advance care planning. Some indi-viduals will not have a loving and knowing relationship, and so, for them, a covenantal relationship may not be achievable or appropriate. Indeed, if we expect advance care planning to be solely covenantal, we would run the risk of setting too high a stan-dard for designating a proxy. This could limit the use of proxies to those who have covenantal relationships.

This is not my objective. My goal is not to restrict proxy desig-nations, but to improve the overall quality of care. We should not require that the relationship transcend the contractual model, but that patients and their proxies aspire toward the covenantal model when it is within reach.

Weighing the benefits and burdens of a contractual or covenantal understanding of the patient-proxy relationship suggests that we need to consider this relationship as having both elements. The mix will be determined by the nature of the relationship that gave birth to the proxy's designation and the clinical circumstances that the proxy ultimately confronts.

It would be a mistake to view this relationship as an either-or proposition that would compel us to choose between a contractual or covenantal framework. Rather, it is best to see the value of bringing both conceptualizations into our deliberations about the legal scope of the proxy's role and the proxy's underlying moral authority. If we can achieve this balance, then our living and dying will be marked by fidelity, wisdom, and love.

NOTES

1. P. Hallie, "An apology to my mother," in P Hallie, *Tales of Good and Evil, Help and Harm* (New York: HarperCollins, 1997), p. 85.

2. By proxy, I mean a surrogate specifically designated by the patient for healthcare decisions while the patient had decision-making capacity. In some jurisdictions, this individual may be known as a durable power of attorney for healthcare or as a healthcare agent.

3. Introducing the notion of covenant into a discussion concerning the relationships that emerge through the use of advance directives is not without some weighty precedents in other areas of medicine. See D. A. Landis, "Physician distinguish thyself: Conflict and covenant in a physician's moral development," *Perspectives in Biology & Medicine* 36 (1993): 628–41; R. Crawshaw et al., "Patient-physician covenant," *JAMA* 273 (1995): 1553; and C. K. Cassel, "The patient-physician covenant: An affirmation of Asklepios," *Ann Int Med* 124 (1996): 604–606.

4. See, for example, President's Commission for the Study of Ethical Problems in Medicine and Biomedical and Behavioral Research, *Deciding to Forgo Life-Sustaining Therapy* (Washington, D.C.: U.S. Government

Printing Office, 1983); A. E. Buchanan and D. W. Brock, *Deciding for Others: The Ethics of Surrogate Decision Making* (New York: Cambridge University Press, 1990), pp. 15–211; New York State Task Force on Life and the Law, *When Others Must Choose: Deciding for Patients without Capacity* (New York: New York State Task Force on Life and the Law, 1992), pp. 47–69; and G. A. Sachs and M. Siegler, "Guidelines for decision making when the patient is incompetent," *J Crit Care Illness* 6 (1991): 348–59.

5. See S. M. Wolf et al., "Sources of concern about the patient self-determination act," *N Engl J Med* 325 (1991): 1666–71.

6. See J. J. Fins, M. D. Bacchetta, and F. G. Miller, "Clinical pragmatism: A method of moral problem solving," *Kennedy Institute of Ethics Journal* 7 (1997): 129–45; and J. J. Fins, F. G. Miller, and M. D. Bacchetta, "Clinical pragmatism: Bridging theory and practice," *Kennedy Institute of Ethics Journal* 8 (1998): 39–44.

7. *The New Shorter Oxford English Dictionary* (Oxford: Clarendon Press, 1993), pp. 496, 534.

8. P. Hallie, "Afterward," in Hallie, *Tales of Good and Evil, Help and Harm,* pp. 209–18.

9. P. Hallie, *Lest Innocent Blood Be Shed* (New York: Harper & Row, 1979); and J. J. Fins, "From indifference to goodness," *Journal of Religion and Health* 35 (1996): 245–54.

10. W. F. May, *Testing the Medical Covenant* (Grand Rapids: W.B. Eerdmans, 1996).

11. W. F. May, "Code and covenant or philanthropy and contract?" in *On Moral Medicine: Theological Perspectives in Medical Ethics,* ed. S. E. Lammers and A. Verhey (Grand Rapids: W. B. Eerdmans, 1987), p. 93.

12. W. F. May, *The Physician's Covenant: Images of the Healer in Medical Ethics* (Philadelphia: Westminster Press, 1983), pp. 106–44.

13. W. A. Elwell, ed., *Baker Encyclopedia of the Bible,* vol. 1 (Grand Rapids: Baker Book House, 1998), pp. 530–38.

God's covenant with Moses also demonstrates that a covenant, unlike a contract, does not necessarily require consent. Although those at Sinai ratified the covenantal relationship in Exodus, in Deuteronomy this covenant was extended to embrace all succeeding generations without their consent: "The Lord our God made a covenant with us at Horeb. It was not with our fathers that the Lord made this covenant, but with us, the living, every one of us who is here today." Deut. 5:2–3. God informs

Moses that, "I make this covenant, with its sanctions, not with you alone, but with those who are standing here with us this day before the Lord our God and with those who are not with us here this day." Deut. 29:13–14.

These passages illustrate another subtle difference between contractual and covenantal relationships. Unlike a contract, a covenant can be something that one does not necessarily choose to do. The covenant between God and his people is an inheritance, with its own set of obligations and responsibilities. Although one can voluntarily enter into such a relationship, one can *be entered* into it as well.

14. Elwell, *Baker Encyclopedia of the Bible*, p. 531.

15. T. M. Knox, ed., *Hegel's Philosophy of Right* (New York: Oxford University Press, 1967), pp. 58, 112.

16. A more recent commentator has suggested how a marriage contract can become covenantal when sanctified by a shared faith: "Without religion, the institution of marriage-the foundation of family life—is no longer the product of vows made solemnly before God; it is just another contract, less binding, even than a mortgage obligation." M. K. Beran, *The Last Patrician: Bobby Kennedy and the End of American Aristocracy* (New York: St. Martin's Press, 1998), p. 182.

17. Having observed that some contractual relationships can evolve into covenantal, it should also be noted that some covenants do not have their origins in contracts.

18. I am indebted to Nancy Dubler for this phrase.

19. N. Dubler and D. Nimmons, *Ethics on Call* (New York: Harmony Books, 1992), pp. 341–65.

20. J. J. Fins, "The Patient Self-Determination Act and patient-physician collaboration in New York State," *New York State Journal of Medicine* 92 (1992): 489–93.

21. New York State Task Force, *When Others Must Choose*, pp. 21–45.

22. A covenantal approach can assist a proxy because it can help him "serve and draw upon the deeper reserves of the other." See May, *The Physician's Covenant*, p. 121.

23. Ibid., p. 119.

24. D. M. High, "Families' roles in advance directives," *Hastings Center Report* 24, no. 6 (1994): S16–S18.

25. P. A. Singer et al., "Reconceptualizing advance care planning from the patient's perspective," *Arch of Int Med* 158 (1997): 879–84.

26. The SUPPORT Investigators, "A controlled trial to improve care for seriously ill hospitalized patients: The study to understand prognoses and preferences for outcomes and risks of treatment (SUPPORT)," *JAMA* 274 (1995): 1591–98.

27. J. M. Teno et al., "Advance directives for seriously ill hospitalized patients: Effectiveness with the Patient Self-determination Act and the SUPPORT intervention," *J Amer Geriat Soc* 45 (1997): 500–507; and J. M. Teno et al., "Do advance directives provide instructions that direct care?" *J Amer Geriatr Soc* 45 (1997): 508–12.

28. J. J. Fins, "Advance directives and SUPPORT," *J Amer Geriatr Soc* 45 (1997): 519–20.

29. J. J. Fins et al., "End-of-life decision-making in the hospital: Current practices and future prospects," *J Pain Symp Mgmt* 17 (1999): 6–15.

21

TWENTY-FIVE YEARS AFTER *QUINLAN*
A Review of the Jurisprudence of Death and Dying

Norman L. Cantor

Since the 1960s, when medical science became capable of prolonging the dying process beyond bounds that many patients
would find acceptable, people have sought "death with dignity,"
or "a natural death," or "a good death." Once debilitation from a
fatal affliction has reached a personally intolerable point, dying
patients have sought to control the manner and timing of death via
diverse techniques. Some sought the disconnection of life-sustaining medical interventions, such as respirators and dialysis
machines. Beyond freedom from unwelcome interventions, some
patients intent on avoiding suffering sought access to pain relief
medication—even in dosages posing some risk (perhaps even a
certainty) of hastening death. Other dying patients sought access
to deep sedation, even knowing that they would never emerge
from the resultant unconsciousness. Still other patients voluntarily
refused to eat or drink or to accept artificial nutrition and hydra-

Reprinted from *Journal of Law, Medicine & Ethics* 29, no. 2 (summer 2001): 182–96, with the
permission of the American Society of Law, Medicine & Ethics. Copyright © 2001. All rights
reserved.

tion. Finally, some sought the more expeditious route of assisted suicide (via a prescription of lethal medication) or even active euthanasia (via a lethal injection at a physician's hand).

From the outset, a variety of forces have sought to circumscribe the human wish to shape one's own dying process. Some religious sources opposed giving a patient the prerogative to control the timing of death on the grounds that only God should have dominion over life and death. Some medical practitioners resisted giving patients this decision-making authority because of professional ideals about preserving human life or a conviction that medical professionals are better suited to making end-of-life decisions than distraught patients or families. Some social observers invoked sanctity of life as a sacrosanct principle and viewed life-shortening measures as inconsistent with that principle. Other observers feared exploitation of vulnerable populations if life-and-death decisions were allocated either to stricken patients or their surrogates. Advocates for disabled persons resented the distasteful message supposedly being broadcast when an afflicted person ended life support on the basis that his or her debilitated existence was intolerable.

Starting in 1976, with the *Quinlan* case in New Jersey,[1] courts and legislatures have outlined the legal bounds governing medical conduct vis-à-vis the dying process. Certain principles have become hallmarks of death and dying jurisprudence. Competent persons have a broad legal prerogative to decide how to respond to fatal afflictions—how much to struggle, how much to suffer, how much bodily invasion to tolerate, and how much helplessness and indignity to endure. They can resist life-sustaining medical interventions even if that step will precipitate their deaths and even if the personal values underlying the choice seem idiosyncratic or foolish. A fatally stricken patient who is unavoidably dying is also probably entitled to stop eating and drinking and to resist artificial nutrition and hydration. Suffering patients are entitled to adequate pain relief medication as part of good palliative care, even if such medication poses a risk of hastening death. And palliative care options should include deep sedation, though the legal status of deep sedation combined with rejection of artificial nutrition and hydration is, for reasons to be explained, still unclear. Active euthanasia and assistance committing suicide are still forbidden, except for Oregon's authorization of physician-assisted suicide.

Even after competence is lost, conscientious surrogates may exercise end-of-life options on behalf of the formerly competent patient. Most legal standards governing surrogate decision making seek to respect the formerly competent patient's self-determination interest by dictating that the surrogate follow the medical course that the patient would presumably want followed. This policy is clearest where the patient has left explicit instructions. In every jurisdiction, for example, a conscientious surrogate can seek an end to artificial life support where the now-incompetent patient previously expressed a desire to reject life support in the situation now at hand. Fulfilling the patient's actual or putative wishes also is the underlying object in jurisdictions employing a substituted judgment standard (replicating what the now-incompetent patient would have wanted done if he or she were miraculously aware of the circumstances at hand). As will be explained, it is also the underlying object in jurisdictions articulating a best-interests standard (asking whether the burdens of continued existence so outweigh the benefits that death can fairly be deemed to be in the patient's best interest). A small number of jurisdictions take a more restrictive approach—precluding removal of life support for a now-incompetent patient absent clear prior expressions that he or she had wanted such a nontreatment course.

This review traces the contours of permissible medical responses to the dying patient's pursuit of death with dignity. The review shows how far death and dying jurisprudence has evolved since *Quinlan*, particularly as to the end-of-life options open to competent patients seeking either to hasten death or to secure palliative relief from suffering. On the other hand, the medical fate of incompetent patients who are dying is far more confused. Jurisdictions vary greatly in the end-of-life options legally available to surrogates acting on behalf of such patients.

COMPETENT PATIENTS

The Legal Foundation

In 1976, *Quinlan* set the pattern for succeeding death and dying jurisprudence. Karen Ann Quinlan was twenty-one years old when a mix of alcohol and drugs caused brain damage, leaving her in a permanently unconscious state. Her biologic functions were maintained by a respirator and artificial nutrition and hydration. Her devoted father sought judicial appointment to be Karen's legal guardian with authority to remove the respirator. Opposition to the father's petition was grounded primarily on claims that detachment of the respirator would constitute murder and that courts should not interfere with her physician's professional judgment in favor of continued life support.

The New Jersey Supreme Court unanimously upheld the father's petition. The court posited that Karen, if competent, would be constitutionally entitled to resist life-sustaining medical intervention. Her entitlement flowed from the Fourteenth Amendment to the U.S. Constitution and its protection of liberty. In light of Karen's incompetence, her loving father should be permitted to exercise this liberty right on his daughter's behalf; otherwise, her constitutional interests (in determining whether to accept life-sustaining medical interventions) would go unprotected. The court repudiated any notions of murder or improper interference with medical judgment. According to the court, the implementation of a patient's constitutional entitlement to resist life-sustaining medical intervention could not be deemed unlawful homicide.

Improper interference with medical judgment was not involved because medical ethics recognized patients' entitlement to choose their own course of treatment (and to have a surrogate choose once the patient had become incapacitated).

Since *Quinlan*, courts have accepted the case's premise that a competent patient may reject life-sustaining medical intervention. A number of state courts echoed *Quinlan* and grounded the patient's prerogative to reject life-sustaining medical intervention in the constitutional protection of liberty.[2] Other courts stressed a nonconstitutional basis—the common law principle that a medical practitioner must secure informed consent before initiating medical treatment.[3] To treat without such consent would be a tort, an unconsented touching. Still other courts used both the Constitution and the common law as the legal foundation for the patient's prerogative. A strong majority of jurisdictions has case law upholding a competent individual's rejection of artificial life support.

In 1990, the U.S. Supreme Court reinforced the notion that the Constitution's protection of liberty encompasses rejection of life-sustaining medical intervention. In the context of a permanently unconscious patient, the Supreme Court noted that many state courts had upheld a patient's prerogative (implemented by a surrogate) to reject treatment and the Court "assumed" for the sake of argument that a *competent* patient would have a constitutional right to reject treatment.[4] Further, the Court followed state court precedents in assuming that the patient could resist artificial nutrition and hydration as well as other forms of medical treatment. Seven years later, the U.S. Supreme Court reaffirmed patients' constitutional right to reject life-sustaining medical intervention, but refused to extend patients' protected options to include ingestion of a poison, i.e., assisted suicide.[5] This 1997 decision focused on the patient's liberty interest in bodily integrity—meaning freedom from unwanted bodily invasions, as opposed to a broader prerogative to control the manner and timing of death.

State court decisions upholding a competent patient's liberty to reject life support have relied on both bodily integrity and patient autonomy—i.e., self-determination in deciding how and if to respond to a fatal affliction.[6] The autonomy interest has prevailed even when the prospective bodily invasions have been rather slight, as in the case of refusal of a life-sustaining blood transfusion.[7] These same decisions have considered and rejected possible governmental interests opposing the patient's prerogative. The cases acknowledge a legitimate governmental interest in promoting sanctity of human life, but they also tend to find that a patient's liberty interests (self-determination and bodily integrity) simply outweigh the state's abstract interest in sanctity of life.[8] The courts note that upholding a dying patient's decision to reject treatment exalts self-determination rather than deprecating sanctity of life. Similarly, courts acknowledge a legitimate government interest in preventing suicide, but refuse to equate rejection of treatment with suicide.[9] The main distinction is that suicide involves initiation of a self-destructive course (e.g., ingesting a poison or shooting oneself), while refusal of treatment involves letting a fatal affliction follow its natural course. Sometimes, there is also a state-of-mind distinction between suicide and rejection of life support. That is, a patient rejecting medical intervention may not desire to die, but to avoid an offensive bodily invasion. This state-of-mind distinction does not always hold up, as some patients rejecting treatment find their quality of life intolerable and indeed wish to die.

Courts have ruled that other conflicting government interests fail to override the competent patient's prerogative to refuse treatment. Efforts to assert a countervailing government interest in upholding medical judgment and medical ethics have met the same fate as in *Quinlan*—a finding that professional ethics recognizes a patient's prerogative to determine his or her medical handling. While the courts acknowledge a healthcare provider's interest in maintaining personal scruples or following one's conscience, the judicial solution is to allow the provider asserting a conscientious objection to refer the patient to another provider and withdraw from the case, thus not overriding the patient's preference to forgo treatment.[10]

Occasionally, the government has asserted an interest in protecting the lives and well-being of dependents of the patient rejecting life support. In at least one early case, in 1964, a court used that rationale to help justify its authorization of medical intervention against a patient's wishes.[11] The court cited the patient's potential "abandonment" of her minor child as one basis for allowing physicians to override the patient's objection to a life-saving blood transfusion. More recent cases have gone the other way, upholding the patient's decision to reject life support as long as the dependents will not be totally abandoned, i.e., there will be a surviving spouse or relative to care for the dependents.[12]

SCOPE OF THE COMPETENT PATIENT'S PREROGATIVE

Types of Medical Interventions, Proximity of Death

Early discussions of a patient's right to reject life-sustaining medical intervention considered possible limitations on that prerogative. One notion was that "extraordinary," but not "ordinary," medical means could be withdrawn at a patient's behest. That dichotomy originated in Roman Catholic doctrine defining "extraordinary" as particularly complex, invasive, or expensive treatments. Under such a framework, a respirator would be deemed extraordinary and therefore expendable, but a blood transfusion would not. The extraordinary/ordinary distinction has not prevailed in legal doctrine. A patient's right to resist bodily invasions encompasses all medical techniques from the simplest aspirin tablet to the most elaborate machine.

In the early 1980s, some commentators sought to differentiate among medical interventions and to exclude the withholding of artificial nutrition and hydration as a medical option.[13] Their contention was that the provision of artificial nutrition and hydration constituted feeding, and that such feeding reflected a basic human obligation and symbolized the nurturing spirit of medicine. The courts have almost uniformly rejected this contention,[14] reasoning that the need for artificial nutrition and hydration is prompted by disease or other pathology and that the patient is entitled to control their provision just as with any other medical response to bodily dysfunction. Some state legislatures, usually in the context of regulating advance medical directives, have been more sympathetic with the effort to distinguish artificial nutrition and hydration from other medical means. This sympathy, though, has only generated a requirement in several states that the declarant specifically mention in the advance directive artificial nutrition and hydration if the declarant wants to reject such treatment. The vast majority of jurisdictions still allow rejection of artificial nutrition and hydration, most of them without a requirement that this rejection be specifically enumerated.

Early cases also hinted that a patient's prerogative to reject treatment might be confined to end-stage care, i.e., when unavoidable death is near at hand. These cases suggested that the government interest in preserving life might prevail against the patient's autonomy interest *unless* life could be only temporarily sustained—when "the issue is not whether, but when, for how long and at what cost to the individual his life may be briefly extended."[15] More recent cases clarify that the patient's prerogative to resist medical intervention is not confined to the end stage of the dying process or even to unavoidably terminal conditions.[16] This means that patients can refuse treatment even at an early stage of a degenerative disease process and, sometimes, in situations where the patients are salvageable to a healthful existence. (This last situation occurs primarily when a patient for religious reasons declines a potentially life-saving medical intervention).

An interesting variation on the right to refuse life-sustaining medical intervention occurs when a dying patient voluntarily stops eating and drinking and declines artificial nutrition and hydration. For a person mired in a prolonged and distasteful degenerative dying process, but not yet machine dependent, the prospect of slipping into a coma and dying of dehydration within fourteen days may seem like an expeditious path to relief. Because the patient who voluntarily stops eating and drinking initiates the cause of death by refusing to ingest, and because the patient is seeking to die, this fatal course of conduct raises the specter of suicide. That specter in turn raises the question of whether medical personnel can legally cooperate with this patient.

Legal precedent on this issue is sparse. Cases dealing with prisoners conducting a hunger strike offer mixed signals, with a few courts upholding a competent prisoner's right to reject artificial nutrition and hydration and the rest finding the conduct a form of suicide and therefore unprotected.[17] Some commentators assert that a patient who has voluntarily stopped eating and drinking has a right to reject artificial nutrition and hydration, and I tend to agree. In contrast to the healthy prisoner initiating a hunger strike, the typical patient who has stopped eating and drinking is acting out of self-determination in response to a fatal affliction. The patient's claim is also reinforced by an interest in bodily integrity (avoiding artificial nutrition and hydration) as well as by general revulsion at the inhumane prospect of restraining or force-feeding a suffering, dying person. These elements will likely override any temptation to label the patient's rejection of nutrition as suicide, even if the patient is purposefully seeking to die. A cooperating physician is then only fulfilling a duty to provide palliative care for a dying patient and is not unlawfully assisting a suicide.[18] In line with this analysis, a couple of trial court judges have refused authorization to force-feed dying elderly patients who had voluntarily stopped eating and drinking.[19]

Note that cardiopulmonary resuscitation (CPR) is governed by principles similar to those applicable to other forms of life-sustaining medical intervention.[20] That is, a competent patient is entitled to dictate that CPR not be performed in the event of cardiac or respiratory arrest. Most hospitals have protocols for obtaining a debilitated patient's (or, where appropriate, a surrogate's) consent to a do-not-resuscitate (DNR) order that is then entered in the patient's chart and signaled to medical personnel in some other fashion. Many states have also adopted protocols for honoring DNR orders in out-of-hospital settings. Medical personnel may also refrain from performing CPR where such intervention is highly unlikely to restore continuous cardiorespiratory function.

Medical Futility

That a competent patient has the right to reject proffered medical treatment does not mean that the patient is similarly entitled to demand treatment not offered. The term "medical futility" has been used to suggest an ultimate limitation on what services patients can demand. The term has aroused considerable dispute. Some sources assert a general medical prerogative to refuse to offer or supply services that are "not medically indicated" or "futile."[21] Other sources view the concept of medical futility as an attempt to reassert provider control over medical services and to undermine the patient's prerogative to shape his or her medical care.[22]

The issue of medical futility is complex. A healthcare provider may legitimately assert a prerogative to assess the physiological utility of possible treatments. That is, a physician's professional judgment includes an assessment of the potential effectiveness of a treatment modality, including the conclusion that it will not have any impact on the patient. A conclusion of physiological futility permits a physician to withhold the treatment modality, subject only to two constraints. To avoid malpractice, the physician must meet professional standards of skill in judging treatment effects.[23] Second, the physician ought to inform the patient about the treatment modality and the physician's judgment of futility; this way the patient has an opportunity to obtain a second opinion.

Where the issue is not physiological futility, but rather the appropriateness of sustaining a severely deteriorated life, the scope of professional judgment is limited. Whether the quality of a patient's remaining existence warrants continued medical treatment is largely a value judgment reserved for the competent patient or the patient's representatives (in conjunction with medical staff) and is not an area for unilateral medical judgment.[24] A healthcare provider in an institutional context can ask for an ethics consultation in the hope of clarifying the medical picture and inducing the patient or representative to alter the course of medical treatment or consent to a cessation of treatment altogether. Also, a healthcare provider may voice conscientious objections to continued medical intervention and may seek to withdraw from the case, provided there is a referral to a more cooperative clinician. But the provider cannot unilaterally terminate life support for a deteriorated, but preservable patient.

Very few cases speak to the concept of medical futility, especially in its qualitative sense involving a judgment that the patient's remaining existence is not worth preserving. In a well-known Minnesota case, a hospital went to court seeking a change of guardian when a husband insisted on continued respirator support for his permanently unconscious spouse.[25] The judge refused to oust the husband as guardian—since the husband purported to be implementing his wife's wishes—and the life support continued. In a Massachusetts case, the daughter of an elderly deceased patient sued Massachusetts General Hospital for having disconnected life support from the then-comatose patient in contravention of the daughter's instructions. In that instance, the attending physician had secured an ethics consultation and received an endorsement from the head of the hospital's ethics committee for removal of life support. A jury refused to award damages against the hospital.[26] Finally, an intermediate appellate court in Louisiana asserted that a physician's liability for unilateral removal of life support from a comatose patient would depend on whether the physician deviated from the prevailing standards of medical practice.[27]

Neither the Massachusetts jury verdict nor the Louisiana judges' position represents a general legal acceptance of a medical prerogative to unilaterally determine qualitative futility. Other cases have imposed liability on hospitals that ended life support for incompetent, debilitated patients in contravention of their surrogates' wishes.[28] Moreover, when a hospital sought judicial authorization to withhold "futile" treatment to an anencephalic infant over the mother's objections, the court declared that the hospital's failure to provide the requested life-extending services would violate a federal statute requiring stabilizing treatment for any emergency medical condition.[29] In sum, a healthcare provider can only hope to invoke the futility concept and overturn a conscientious surrogate's insistence on continued life support when the surrogate's course is abusive—i.e., when the patient is being subjected to pointless suffering or when the surrogate's course is inexplicably aberrant from what the vast majority of people would want.

Palliative Care: Risky Analgesics to Terminal Sedation

Provision of effective pain relief is increasingly viewed as an integral part of medical responsibility to patients.[30] In recent years, the medical profession has moved rapidly to increase education about pain control, to establish guidelines for practitioners engaged in treating intractable pain, and to eliminate perceived barriers to the use of opioids as part of palliative care. This increased sensitivity to palliative care comes in reaction to two phenomena—studies showing that a high percentage of dying patients experience significant pain despite major advances in analgesic techniques, and claims by some sources that unrelieved suffering of some dying patients necessitates resorting to physician-assisted suicide.

From a legal perspective, there is no question that healthcare providers are allowed to furnish effective analgesic relief even when the pain medication poses some risk of hastening a patient's death. The professional imperative to mitigate suffering justifies some risk of hastening death. The matter is analogous to a risky open-heart surgery; the prospect of a patient's major gain in quality of life justifies the risk involved in the surgery. Of course, professional guidelines exist for administering pain relief, and healthcare providers must conform to them in order to avoid malpractice liability or professional discipline. These guidelines require that any risky pain relief be necessary—i.e., that the pain be intractable; that less dangerous, but effective analgesics do not exist; and that the dosage be titrated upward in a careful fashion.

The conventional wisdom in medicolegal circles says that a healthcare provider can lawfully give a risky dose of analgesics as long as the impetus is a patient's severe suffering and the provider's specific intention is to ease suffering rather than to cause death. The New York State Task Force on Life and the Law observed:

> It is widely recognized that the provision of pain medication is ethically and professionally acceptable even when the treatment may hasten the patient's death if the medication is intended to alleviate pain and severe discomfort, not to cause death.[31]

This focus on the provider's intention in administering palliative care seeks to transpose the doctrine of double effect to the medicolegal context.[32] Under that doctrine, a proportionately good effect (relief of suffering) may overcome a foreseeable bad effect (causing death) as long as the doctor does not intend to accomplish the bad effect. The effort to use the doctrine of double effect, with its focus on a physician's intention, seems inconsistent with traditional legal doctrine, which establishes that it is criminal homicide to knowingly cause death, even if the doctor's motive or intention is to relieve suffering. Mercy killing has always been prohibited in the Anglo-American system. Thus, at least if an analgesic dosage is certain or practically certain to hasten death, the physician's knowing conduct constitutes an unlawful killing closely akin to active euthanasia.[33]

In the 1997 cases rejecting constitutional challenges to state bans on physician-assisted suicide, the Supreme Court apparently accepted the conventional wisdom about aggressive palliative care with its focus on a palliative caregiver's intention.[34] Chief Justice Rehnquist's opinion on behalf of five justices approvingly referred to the availability of pain relief that might hasten death as long as "the medication is intended to alleviate pain and some discomfort, not to cause death."[35] Some concurring justices went even further in assuming that state law commonly allows administration of pain relief medication even in dosages that the physician knows will hasten death (as opposed to merely incurring a risk that death will be hastened).[36] These expressions, however, are in tension with the traditional criminal law principle that to knowingly cause death is a form of unlawful homicide.

The better explanation for the legality of aggressive palliative care is found in criminal law principles of recklessness and justification; these principles allow a measure of medical risk taking short of knowingly causing death. Consequently, a physician is justified in incurring some risk of death (but not a certainty of death) in order to relieve a patient's unbearable suffering.[37] No criminal responsibility is incurred unless the palliative care provider is reckless and grossly departs from professional standards. Current professional standards authorize risky analgesics when they are necessary to relieve intractable suffering. "The risk of death is justified, not because it is unintended but because there is no alternative approach that makes the risk of death less likely and the alleviation of suffering possible."[38] The fact that the physician administering pain relief is creating a risk of death rather than certainly precipitating death also helps differentiate legitimate pain relief from euthanasia. "We view the administration of morphine to reduce suffering not really as killing but as an act of risking death to secure pain relief, analogous to risking death by submitting to a potentially life-saving operation."[39]

Another form of aggressive pain relief is deep sedation, rendering an egregiously suffering, dying patient unconscious or stuporous during the remainder of the dying process. The medical objective is to relieve a variety of intractable physical or emotional conditions sometimes accompanying the dying process. Refractory physical suffering can be engendered by pain or discomforts such as nausea, vomiting, or dyspnea. Emotional suffering can be associated with respiratory distress, agitation, fatigue, incontinence, or helplessness. In the small percentage of cases in which customary palliative care does not adequately relieve suffering, deep sedation becomes a possible course. This is known as terminal sedation, where the patient is likely to expire while still sedated.

Most forms of deep sedation are clearly lawful under the principles of recklessness and justification discussed above. For example, deep sedation is frequently used as an adjunct to withdrawal of life-sustaining medical machinery, such as extubation of a ventilator-dependent patient. To avoid any suggestion of criminality, care providers are expected to use sedative dosages commensurate with keeping the patient unconscious, but not with killing the patient. Any modest risk that the sedatives will hasten death is justified by the need to relieve suffering. The same legal rationale applies to another form of terminal sedation—one used when an egregiously suffering patient is within hours or days of death. Because the patient is near death, it is impossible to know definitively whether the deep sedation hastens death or whether the underlying disease process has taken its toll. But as long as the sedation is administered at a level geared to maintaining unconsciousness, the risk that death might be hastened is justified by the palliative necessity.

A problematic element sometimes connected with deep sedation is the simultaneous withholding of artificial nutrition and hydration. Some commentators contend that this cessation serves as a gratuitous means of hastening the sedated patient's death (via dehydration)—a "gratuitous" means assertedly akin to euthanasia because the relief of suffering is already accomplished by deep sedation.[40] The withholding of artificial nutrition and hydration does not seem to pose a serious legal problem in the typical case, where the deep sedation is instituted only during the last few days of the patient's dying process. The patient is already gravely debilitated and may naturally have cut back on food and fluid intake had he or she been conscious; consequently, it would be impossible to establish the withholding of food and fluids on the patient's behalf as the cause of death. Moreover, there is often a palliative justification—such as avoidance of pulmonary edema—for withholding food and fluids as part of end-stage care.

The problematic aspect of terminal sedation surfaces if withholding artificial nutrition and hydration takes place at an earlier point in the dying process, say, many weeks before the patient would have normally died from the underlying disease. In that instance, death from dehydration might plausibly be shown. There is no real legal precedent, so an analysis of the legality of long-term terminal sedation accompanied by a withholding of artificial nutrition and hydration must be tentative.[41] One perspective is that once relief of suffering is achieved via deep sedation, withholding nutrition and fluids has no palliative function and, therefore, risking death by dehydration has no legal justification. As the patient may well intend that the rejection of artificial nutrition and hydration hasten death, overtones of suicide are present. If a healthcare provider contemplating administration of long-term deep sedation knows that the patient also plans to reject artificial nutrition and hydration, initiation of deep sedation knowingly sets in motion a fatal course and might arguably be regarded as facilitation of a suicide—a step raising some ethical, if not legal, qualms.

A contrary perspective is that the patient voluntarily choosing long-term terminal sedation is exercising legitimate prerogatives that the healthcare provider ought to respect. Certainly, deep sedation is a legitimate palliative step. A patient who then resists artificial nutrition and hydration is invoking an important interest in bodily integrity—a prerogative to resist bodily invasions long recognized in death and dying jurisprudence. For example, a dying patient is probably entitled to stop eating and drinking even though he or she is intentionally hastening death. Moreover, a dying patient resisting artificial nutrition and hydration has an important self-determination interest in avoiding the indignity of lingering indefinitely in a deeply sedated state. In a sense, long-term terminal sedation can be regarded as part of a natural dying process—namely, a fatal pathology causes egregious suffering, necessitating deep sedation and that sedation, in turn, shuts down the natural alimentation system. However, the sequence of long-term terminal sedation followed by a withholding of artificial nutrition and hydration is legally uncharted territory. While some concurring justices in *Glucksberg* made favorable reference to the administration of analgesics at levels high enough to cause unconsciousness, for the sake of pain relief, it is doubtful that they were as yet endorsing long-term terminal sedation accompanied by a withholding of artificial nutrition and hydration.

Physician-Assisted Suicide

Advocates of death with dignity are not fully satisfied with the options currently available to dying patients, such as rejection of life-sustaining medical intervention, access to analgesics, voluntary refusal to continue eating or drinking, or terminal sedation (in its clearly lawful forms). Each option usually entails some period of lingering in a highly debilitated or helpless state and, therefore, offends the dignity these advocates are intent on preserving. They therefore push for more expeditious means of hastening death—particularly physician-assisted suicide (giving a competent patient access to a lethal poison).

Only Oregon has legalized physician-assisted suicide. Virtually all the remaining states treat assistance to suicide as a crime, either by statute or by common law. Supporters of physician-assisted suicide have sought to overcome these legal hurdles by popular referendum, legislation, and constitutional attack. Except in Oregon, the referendum/legislative route has thus far failed. Indeed, a significant number of states have in the last several years adopted legislation clarifying or reiterating their opposition to physician-assisted suicide. Nor has the constitutional route succeeded to date. In 1996, two federal courts of appeals upheld constitutional attacks on Washington's and New York's ban on physician-assisted suicide as applied to competent, suffering, terminally ill patients.[42] But in 1997, on appeal to the U.S. Supreme Court, these decisions were overturned. The Supreme Court rejected the constitutional challenges.[43] State courts have similarly rejected constitutional challenges to laws banning physician-assisted suicide.[44]

Proponents contend that physician-assisted suicide—as confined to a suffering, terminally ill patient—is morally and practically indistinguishable from other forms of hastening death that states have accepted. These "other forms" refer to medical withdrawal of life support at the patient's behest and to medical use of risky analgesics or sedatives. The proponents' constitutional attacks have focused on the claimed arbitrariness of state policy in banning physician-assisted suicide while accepting these other forms of hastening death.

With its decisions in 1997, the Supreme Court forcefully repudiated these attacks. Chief Justice Rehnquist's opinion acknowledged a patient's Fourteenth Amendment liberty right to choose death by rejecting life-sustaining medical intervention. But he viewed the constitutional liberty interest in rejecting life support as grounded in bodily integrity rather than autonomy to choose how and when to die. He also saw a rational distinction between rejection of medical intervention and ingestion of a poison. The former involves letting the dying process take its natural course, while the latter involves a self-initiated precipitation of death. (Although a physician's withdrawal of life support is in one sense an action precipitating death, it simply removes previously instituted obstacles to a natural dying process.)

Chief Justice Rehnquist also referred to medical ethics as providing a plausible basis for distinguishing physician-assisted suicide from other forms of hastening death. Many medical professional groups regard assistance in killing—such as the provision of a poison—as incompatible with the traditional medical role of curing and comforting. Finally, Rehnquist perceived certain hazards associated with physician-assisted suicide that would legitimize the prevailing legal ban. The principal hazard cited was abuse of vulnerable populations. Dying patients are notoriously distressed and depressed, subject to influence or manipulation; moreover, elderly and minority patients might be subject to a healthcare provider's prejudice and, therefore, be particularly prone to manipulation.

All these concerns about legalization of physician-assisted suicide are understandable, but highly debatable. The Supreme Court made clear that states are free to resolve the public policy debate either by maintaining the status quo or changing it, as did Oregon. The ultimate direction of public policy is hard to gauge. The killing/letting die distinction used to justify the continuing ban on physician-assisted suicide seems quite fragile. The notion that the ban symbolically reinforces the state's interest in defending and preserving the sanctity of life by narrowly confining the scope of lawful killings is eroded by the public perception that both medical withdrawal of life support and the administration of risky analgesics (in high, probably lethal, dosages) are legally accepted forms of killing.

Medical ethics also provides a fragile foundation for the ban on physician-assisted suicide. Although major professional organizations declare that assistance to suicide is incompatible with the medical role, a large number of healthcare professionals perceive relief of a dying patient's unbearable suffering—even by a poison, if necessary—as consistent with a palliative medical role when curative and restorative measures are no longer realistic.[45]

Fear of abuse of vulnerable populations looms as the most enduring obstacle to legalization of physician-assisted suicide.

However, the purveyors of fear will have to explain why comparable abuses of vulnerable populations have not surfaced in other end-of-life contexts, such as withdrawal of life support and use of risky analgesics. Depression, prejudice, and financial pressure potentially affect removal of life support just as they would affect physician-assisted suicide, yet no widespread abuse of vulnerable populations involving removal of life support has occurred. Experience in Oregon and in the Netherlands will help determine whether the specter of abuse will continue to block the legalization of physician-assisted suicide. It is too early to tell about Oregon, though early reports find no abuse there. The data regarding the Netherlands is controversial, with observers on both sides of the debate finding support for their positions in the Dutch experience.[46]

INCOMPETENT PATIENTS

When the *Quinlan* case was pending in 1976, some commentators issued dire warnings about allowing disconnection of life support from incompetent, helpless persons. The cry was that detaching Karen Ann Quinlan's respirator would constitute murder and that its approval by the courts would lead to involuntary euthanasia of senile and other debilitated human beings. Yet, the New Jersey Supreme Court resisted the *in terrorem* arguments. The court understood that requiring medical maintenance of all incompetent, dying persons, no matter how hopeless and deteriorated their conditions, would entail inhumane and unwanted medical intervention. It ruled that Karen Ann Quinlan, if competent, would have had the right to resist continued life support. In light of her incapacity (permanent unconsciousness), her right could be exercised by a conscientious guardian, such as her loving father. Protection against abuse would be assured by the presence of attending medical personnel and by the scrutiny of a prognosis committee that had to be consulted.

Most jurisdictions have followed the pattern fixed by *Quinlan*. That is, most states allow a conscientious guardian (usually, but not always, a close family member) to make end-of-life medical decisions on behalf of an incompetent, terminally ill patient. As will be explained below, the precise decision-making criteria and procedures vary from state to state. Many of the cases deal with permanently unconscious patients, like Ms. Quinlan, who obviously could not benefit in any meaningful fashion from continued medical intervention. But many cases and statutes deal with—and authorize—withdrawal of life support from some persons still capable of relating to their environment with continued medical intervention. A small number of jurisdictions, fearing exploitation of helpless persons, exclude surrogates from making any decision to end life unless the now-incompetent patient had given clear indication of desiring such a course when he or she was competent.

The starting point of most statutes and cases relating to incompetent, dying patients is to honor prospective autonomy—that is, state law often instructs surrogate decision makers to implement any discernible advance instructions issued by the patient. This respect for the formerly competent patient's wishes pervades the legislation governing advance medical directives and, to a lesser extent, characterizes the case law and statutes applicable when no advance directive has been issued. The details follow.

ADVANCE MEDICAL DIRECTIVES

Every state allows competent persons to dictate in advance how they would like their medical care to be resolved once they become incompetent. One means is appointing a healthcare agent who will be responsible for directing medical personnel once the principal becomes incompetent. (This agent may be known by diverse titles, such as proxy or surrogate.)

Having a healthcare agent, especially one who is familiar with the patient's wishes, has obvious benefits. The agent will be functioning according to up-to-date information about the patient's condition and prognosis, as opposed to written instructions that would only reflect the patient's best guess about circumstances months or years in advance of their occurrence. The agent can also act as an advocate and enforcer of the patient's wishes in the event of resistance from healthcare providers.

The relevant statutes instruct the appointed agent to follow the now-incompetent patient's wishes as reflected in prior expressions or other indicia of the patient's values and preferences regarding end-of-life decisions. In the absence of discernible patient preferences, the agent is generally instructed by statute to follow the patient's best interests.

Regardless of whether a person appoints an agent, he or she can seek to control postcompetence medical intervention by issuing advance instructions, sometimes called an advance directive, instruction directive, or living will. I will use the term *advance directive*.

Some commentators doubt the utility or efficacy of advance directives.[47] At the moment of drafting one, a declarant must anticipate a multitude of possible medical scenarios. Moreover, the declarant must project how he or she will feel in a variety of inherently unknowable incompetent mental states. Some commentators also argue that the values or preferences of a previously competent declarant don't matter once the patient has become gravely debilitated and can't appreciate any deviation from his or her prior instructions.[48]

However, these objections don't obviate the importance of advance directives. While declarants may be unable to anticipate the precise scenario they will face when dying, they may have well-developed and enduring notions of dignity, religion, and consideration for loved ones, which they want reflected in their future medical handling. Personal values and preferences reflected in an advance directive can be important for the sake of self-determination even if the advance directive's violation is never known to its author, given the person's debilitated state when the advance directive comes into play. People, while still competent, care mightily whether their cherished values, including dignity, will ultimately be respected in the dying process. In recognition of the importance of this self-determination, virtually all jurisdictions provide that a person's articulated wishes contained in an advance directive should be honored postcompetence, just as a person's wishes about testamentary disposition of property are respected even though the dead person cannot sense violation of those wishes.

Certain intrinsic difficulties of advance directives preclude their ever being a panacea regarding end-of-life decision making. Perhaps because thinking about the dying process is generally distasteful, only a modest percentage of people (usually estimated at 20 percent) prepare advance directives. Even when an advance directive has been prepared, physicians sometimes insist on following their own treatment preferences rather than those of the declarant, particularly if the physician perceives that the advance instructions conflict with the current best interests of the now-incompetent patient. Sometimes, a designated healthcare agent or other surrogate becomes distraught or guilt-ridden and unable to implement the advance instructions.

Medical uncertainty also poses an unavoidable obstacle to the implementation of an advance directive. A document may provide for cessation of life support when there is no longer a "significant" or "realistic" chance of "recovery"; yet physicians may not be able to say definitively whether the patient will recover or whether any prospective recovery will be accompanied by serious impairments.

The biggest obstacle, however, is the imprecision or vagueness frequently present in advance directives. A common model contains one operative sentence instructing a surrogate decision maker: "If I [the declarant] should be in an incurable or irreversible mental or physical condition with no reasonable expectation of recovery, I direct my attending physician to withhold or withdraw treatment that merely prolongs my dying."[49] Such language is presumably intended to avoid a lingering, undignified demise, but it does not elucidate the particulars of debilitation or indignity that would be intolerable to the declarant. An advance directive ought to provide more meaningful guidance by focusing on the elements of indignity—such as mental deterioration, immobility, or helplessness—that the declarant deems personally intolerable. Certain advance directives specify personally intolerable levels of deterioration.[50] But the bulk of advance directives continue to be vague and uninformative.

Statutes in some jurisdictions purport to limit the effectiveness of advance directives to situations where the patient is in a "terminal condition," variously defined.[51] If strictly applied, such statutory provisions would impede implementation of advance directives at the early stages of degenerative dying processes or where the deteriorated, incompetent patient is maintainable for a substantial period. In most instances, though, the governing statute contains a saving provision saying that the statutory framework does not derogate from the existing common law prerogatives of the declarant. Those common law prerogatives probably encompass a right to dictate in advance the withholding of life-sustaining treatment even if the now-incompetent patient has not yet reached the end stage of a dying process or a statutorily defined "terminal condition."[52]

DECISION-MAKING STANDARDS BINDING SURROGATES

As noted, most people do not provide advance instructions regarding end-of-life medical treatment. The states vary widely in the judicially or statutorily defined standards or criteria that are then supposed to govern a surrogate's decision making on behalf of an incompetent, dying patient. The following material sketches the divergent legal approaches.

Evidence of Previously Expressed Wishes

Courts in a small number of states, most notably Missouri and New York, have ruled that surrogates (aside from designated healthcare agents) can end life support only if the patient previously left clear and convincing evidence that he or she would have wanted that course followed under the circumstance now at hand.[53] Michigan and Wisconsin have a similar policy, at least for dying patients who still have the capacity to relate to their environment—i.e., they are not permanently unconscious.[54] This position—requiring clear and convincing proof of the now-incompetent patient's previously expressed wishes—is grounded in the apprehension that helpless patients would otherwise be abused by insensitive quality-of-life decisions on the part of prejudiced or self-interested decision makers.

The hesitance to empower surrogates is not entirely unfounded. There have been cases where parents and healthcare providers made improper terminal decisions about disabled newborns. Perhaps the most notorious case was *Infant Doe* in 1982, where the parents ordered life-sustaining intervention withheld from a Down's Syndrome newborn because they believed that any such handicapped child would lead an unhappy life.[55]

Although well intended, the requirement of clear and convincing evidence of the now-incompetent patient's wish to withdraw life support represents a harsh and inhumane constraint on end-of-life decision making. Very few people articulate their prospective wishes with the precision demanded by the few courts following this standard. The consequence, under the clear and convincing evidence approach, is that many individuals have been forced to linger in gravely debilitated states (such as permanent unconsciousness), which they would almost surely have wanted to avoid.[56] For the never-competent patient—the person who has always been severely developmentally disabled—the result is presumably that all possible life-maintenance must be continued, as such a person could never have given clear and convincing evidence of a wish to die. Again, the result is harsh, as patients would have to be sustained no matter how much suffering or debilitation was being endured.

Though the clear and convincing standard is harsh and imprudent, it is constitutional. In 1990, the U.S. Supreme Court considered a challenge to the Missouri policy precluding withdrawal of life support absent clear and convincing evidence of previously expressed wishes.[57] The challenge came from parents seeking the removal of a nasogastric tube from their adult daughter who had been reduced to a permanently unconscious state by a traumatic injury. A majority of the Supreme Court ruled that Missouri's approach was constitutionally defensible as a means of protecting helpless, incompetent persons against abuse at the hands of surrogates who might find their continued existence burdensome or inconvenient. Fortunately, the vast majority of jurisdictions trust surrogates, in conjunction with healthcare providers, to make end-of-life medical decisions for incompetent patients even in those situations for which the patients did not clearly articulate their wishes. The alternative approaches used by these jurisdictions follow.

Substituted Judgment

In the mid-seventies to mid-eighties, when death and dying jurisprudence was largely being shaped, a number of courts proclaimed that an incompetent patient should enjoy "the same panoply of rights" as a competent person.[58] This would include the competent patient's right to reject life-sustaining medical intervention. The notion of "the same panoply of rights" honors autonomy by indicating that a person's values and preferences ought to govern medical treatment even after competence is lost. A surrogate can seek to implement the patient's autonomy right by choosing the course that the patient, if able, would have chosen for himself or herself.

Substituted judgment is one name for this decision-making standard that strives to implement the now-incompetent patient's previous wishes or preferences regarding end-of-life treatment. The surrogate decision maker is instructed to replicate what the now-incompetent patient would have chosen if somehow miraculously competent and aware of all the circumstances confronting him or her. A number of jurisdictions have explicitly adopted a substituted judgment approach.[59] Under this approach, the patient's previously expressed wishes or preferences—in the form of an advance directive or some other indicia of preference—would govern the surrogate's decision.

The surrogate's task under the substituted judgment approach may be easy enough when an explicit advance directive exists, the patient has left oral instructions, or the patient adhered to religious or philosophical positions that dictate the course the patient would have taken under the circumstances. The problem occurs in the many instances when the now-incompetent patient has not left clear indicia of end-of-life treatment preferences. Some jurisdictions employ a loose, substituted judgment approach and expect the surrogate to extrapolate the patient's likely choice based on whatever knowledge is available about the patient's previous values and preferences. This approach is especially common when the patient is in a permanently unconscious state.[60] Some commentators are skeptical, however, of a surrogate's capacity to project the now-incompetent patient's likely choice when there were no clear-cut prior expressions regarding end-of-life care. These commentators are fearful that the surrogate will project the surrogate's own values and preferences rather than the patient's.[61]

Many jurisdictions view the subjective or substituted judgment approach—seeking to discern the patient's actual wishes—as only a starting point along the end-of-life decision-making spectrum.[62] If the now-incompetent patient's wishes can be discerned, they should, of course, be followed exactly. In the absence of determinative indicia of the patient's preferences regarding end-of-life treatment, however, the surrogate is expected to shift to a "best interests of the patient" approach.[63] That approach acknowledges the possibility that the burdens of continued existence might out-weigh its benefits, i.e., that the incompetent patient might be better off dead than alive. This standard has its own difficulties, now to be considered.

Best Interests of the Patient

While public policy respects autonomous choice, oftentimes a now-incompetent patient's actual preferences about end-of-life treatment cannot be reliably determined. Many jurisdictions—either by statute or case law—then prescribe that the patient's best interests should guide the surrogate's decision making on behalf of the incompetent patient. The best-interests approach is sup-posed to be an objective standard geared to promoting the patient's well-being.

Well-being usually means continued existence. Yet, in the con-text of close-to-death decisions, the burdens of continued existence may, sometimes, be judged to outweigh its benefits—that is, the incompetent patient may sometimes be deemed better off dead than alive. In those instances, surrogates may, consistent with the best-interests approach, seek a removal of life support. This approach sounds simple enough, but significant difficulties occur either in defining the patient's burdens or in measuring them vis-à-vis the benefits of continued living.

The overall object of the best-interests standard is to treat people the way they would want to be treated and, in the absence of definitive indicia of their actual preferences, the assumption is that incapacitated patients want to be treated the way most people would want to be treated under the circumstances. This overall approach helps define the components of the best-interests stan-dard—the burdens and benefits of continued existence for the patient. These components are formulated according to the perceptions of what the average person (sometimes known as the reasonable person) would deem to be critical factors in end-of-life decision making.[64] This means a starting presumption in favor of maintenance of life (as most people, even those grievously ill, want to keep living) and an accompanying principle that extreme suffering is intolerable (given people's common aversion to extreme pain). The process from there is to implement the patient's *likely* choice by having the surrogate act according to the factors and criteria most people would choose for themselves, though it should be kept in mind that this approach does not ignore the patient's personal preferences. Any discernible, competently expressed wishes should take precedence in governing the patient's medical fate either because an inquiry into the patient's subjective preferences precedes resorting to the best-interests standard or because a person's self-defined best interests count in the best-interests calculus.

While severe suffering is a relevant burden to be considered in any best-interests approach, assessing that burden can be a daunting task. In many instances, the extreme debilitation of the incompetent patient prevents any effective communication about feelings and, therefore, impedes understanding the patient's experiential reality. Those surrounding the dying patient must then struggle to interpret cryptic clues—enigmatic sounds, gestures, facial expressions, and nonverbal behavior.[65] Do moans and tugging at tubes reflect unbearable suffering or just a reflexive response to an annoyance? Does a smile reflect pleasure or just gratitude for a kind, but futile, gesture by a care provider? To what extent does the patient's incomprehension increase the anxiety and fear accompanying medical interventions? In short, problems of interpretation plague any surrogate seeking to determine an incompetent patient's level of suffering, or the relative weights to give the patient's suffering and satisfaction. "The real burdens and benefits of life in extremely debilitating circumstances are often beyond our ability to know confidently or comprehend fully."[66]

Uncertainty about the component elements of one's best interests also plagues application of the standard. A prime example is the well-being of the incompetent patient's surrounding loved ones. Can the surrogate consider the emotional and financial impact on the patient's loved ones in fixing the medical course to be followed? One perspective is that most people would include their loved ones' emotional and financial well-being in defining their own best interests in end-of-life situations.[67] Most people do not want to become a burden to their families and, therefore, want the effect of their medical care on their loved ones to be considered. Accordingly, a few cases mention family interests as a legitimate factor in the best-interests calculus.[68]

A contrary perspective is that by injecting nonpatients' interests into the decision-making process, the surrogate is unfairly balancing the value of one person's life against the necessarily secondary impact on others. This kind of utilitarian calculus has always been anathema in the context of individual end-of-life decision making, due both to the incommensurability of a life contrasted with other people's burdens and to societal revulsion toward Nazi efforts to apply a utilitarian calculus to helpless medical patients.

An alternative, intermediate approach to considering or not considering family interests would be to allow consideration of family or caregiver interests only if the patient stipulated that such factors be considered or if the patient's consistently expressed values embraced such an altruistic approach. In the meantime, no legal consensus exists regarding the role of family interests within the best-interests formula.

Another controversial component of the best-interests formula is the patient's quality of life. The 1983 President's Commission listed "quality as well as the extent of life sustained" as a major element of the best-interests standard.[69] This is fully consistent with the underlying object of identifying factors that a reasonable person would deem to be part of his or her best interests. Most people care mightily about what their quality of life may be should they become incompetent or, in particular, suffer extreme mental deterioration before dying.[70]

Not surprisingly, courts that embrace a best-interests standard frequently mention quality-of-life factors, such as loss of function, humiliation, dependence, and loss of dignity, as relevant considerations for a surrogate.[71] These decisions implicitly recognize that, at some level of physical and mental deterioration, the patient's life becomes so demeaning and distasteful that continued existence, for the reasonable person anyway, becomes worse than nonexistence.

Some commentators criticize using quality of life as a factor when applying the best-interests standard. They regard quality of life as an imprecise, value-laden notion lacking a consistent content and subject to exploitation by surrogates indifferent or hostile to the fate of debilitated, vulnerable patients. This concern is, in large part, responsible for the narrow approach that prevails in New York and a few other jurisdictions (i.e., the clear and convincing evidence of previously expressed wishes standard).

An alternative to adopting a narrower standard, though, is an approach that acknowledges people's common preoccupation with dignity in end-of-life care and recognizes the difficulty of assessing the current feelings of deeply demented patients, yet precludes arbitrary or abusive quality-of-life determinations by surrogates.

Constructive Preference

There is a surrogate decision-making standard—one I call "constructive preference"—that promotes the central mission of both the substituted judgment and best-interests formulae (that is, replication of what the now-incompetent patient would have wanted done in the circumstances confronting him or her).[72] The premise of the constructive-preference standard is that the vast majority of people care about indignity or quality of life in the dying process, and that common preferences about intolerable levels of indignity can be ascertained and used to guide surrogate decision makers. At least regarding certain commonly occurring end-of-life scenarios, strong majority preferences can be objectively determined and used as default presumptions (in the absence of actual, competently expressed preferences) to guide surrogates. While "constructive preference" is my own term, several courts do recognize the relevance of most people's end-of-life preferences in shaping surrogate decision making on behalf of now-incompetent patients who have left no clear instructions.[73]

The societal importance of avoiding indignity in the dying process is patent. People fear that grave debilitation will entail embarrassment and/or frustration stemming from helplessness, dependence, and incapacity. Even if these distasteful feelings do not materialize, people care about the images and recollections they will leave behind—they may not want their loved ones' memories of them to be forever sullied by images of extreme mental and physical deterioration during the dying process. These common preoccupations with avoiding indignity before death are readily observable in the context of competent patients contemplating their prospective medical fates—specifically, in decisions to reject life-sustaining medical intervention, in advance medical directives, and in attitudinal surveys showing "paramount importance [attached to] . . . functional independence and the maintenance of mental faculties."[74]

Of course, many commentators express concern about the possible imprecision and subjectivity of the dignity concept in end-of-life decision making. Sanford Kadish remarks: "[T]he difficulty is that we have no way to make confident judgments about how far cognitive and physical deterioration must go before life ceases to be worth living, because the value judgments implicit in such a conclusion are in sharp contention in our society."[75] To avoid arbitrariness and abuse, then, dignity-based guidelines must be grounded in reliable measures of what most people would deem to be intolerable indignity for themselves in the dying process.

The tools exist for assessing common attitudes about indignity in the dying process. Two primary sources of data about competent persons' preferences regarding their own medical fates are advance medical directives (viewed in bulk) and surveys regarding prospective medical handling. Some advance directives—particularly those in which declarants have completed a values profile—communicate their authors' visions of intolerable indignity in the dying process.[76] Many surveys scrutinize people's preferences regarding end-of-life decisions and highlight attitudes toward elements of indignity often encountered in dying patients, such as the incapacity to feed or dress oneself, incontinence, and severe dementia. These sources can provide definitive guidance as to what the prevailing attitudes are toward certain commonly confronted end-of-life scenarios. These data can also be supplemented by healthcare providers' observations regarding widespread patient preferences.

Some implications of a constructive-preference approach to surrogate decision making are apparent. For example, permanent unconsciousness is an intolerably undignified status under contemporary societal standards. Public surveys, judicial decisions upholding a surrogate's decision to terminate life support, and legislative enactments all confirm that indefinite maintenance in a permanently insensate, immobile state is intolerably demeaning to the vast majority of people contemplating their own medical fates. Because of this overwhelming majority sentiment, the presumption under a constructive-preference standard would be that a permanently unconscious patient would prefer death to an existence devoid of all sensation or feeling.[77] A surrogate would be expected to seek removal of life support from any such patient unless the surrogate presented significant evidence that the particular patient deviated from the strong majority sentiment about permanent unconsciousness.

A similar presumption might ultimately be extended to dying persons who are conscious, but so demented as to be unable to recognize and relate to other people. Many people regard such an existence as intolerably undignified for themselves. If ongoing inquiry determines that a strong majority of persons share that sentiment, then a surrogate would be expected to allow a patient in that grievously demented condition to expire without further medical intervention (absent significant evidence that the particular patient deviated from the strong majority sentiment). Conceivably, inquiry might reveal that a substantial percentage (say, 50 to 70 percent, but less than a strong majority) of people regard this profoundly demented state as intolerably undignified for themselves. In that instance, a surrogate should probably have discretion, but not a duty, to seek removal of further life-sustaining medical intervention. Courts or legislatures in each jurisdiction would ultimately have to define the bounds of "strong majority" and "substantial percentage."

The constructive preferences to be used in applying the standard would evolve over time as more data become available about people's end-of-life preferences. Regardless of this evolution, though, the approach would apply only to previously competent persons who had never provided explicit guidance or clear-cut indications about the end-of-life treatment they desired. As to such patients, it makes sense to ascertain what most people would want in similar circumstances and to treat the now-incompetent patients accordingly. As long as the constructive preferences (i.e., the default presumptions) are anchored in objective data concerning what competent people would consider an intolerably undignified existence for themselves, the standard would effectively restrain surrogates' arbitrary or subjective visions of what lives are worth preserving.

CONCLUSION

Death and dying jurisprudence since *Quinlan* presents either a glass that is half full or half empty, depending on your perspective.

Looking first at the full portion, we should appreciate that American jurisprudence permits a number of ways in which a competent patient can avoid a prolonged dying process plagued by either extreme suffering or debilitation to the point of intolerable indignity. The law acknowledges a medical patient's prerogative—grounded in self-determination and bodily integrity—to reject life-sustaining medical interventions. This prerogative attaches no matter how slight the bodily intrusions contemplated, no matter how long the patient's existence could potentially be preserved, and no matter how foolish the patient's decision might seem to health-care providers and others. Moreover, the competent, dying patient is probably entitled to accelerate the dying process by refusing to eat or drink. There also is a possibility that in cases of extreme suffering a patient would be entitled to seek deep sedation accompanied by a withholding of artificial nutrition and hydration—a technique ensuring death within a few weeks. In any event, the patient is always entitled to effective palliative care including, if necessary, pain relief medication in dosages that risk hastening death.

Also favoring the half-full view of the glass, the law accepts prospective autonomy—namely, a person's prerogative to determine his or her postcompetence medical handling by appointing a healthcare agent in advance or by dictating advance instructions, or both. Even in the absence of advance planning of this sort, most jurisdictions allow a surrogate to shape end-of-life medical care on behalf of a now-incompetent patient. The surrogate can determine, in conjunction with medical staff, either that the patient would not—if capable of deciding for himself or herself—want life support continued, or that life support should be discontinued because the burdens of continued existence outweigh any potential benefits. This deference to surrogate choice is particularly prevalent when the patient has reached a permanently unconscious state. (This deference, though, reflects more a recognition of the intrinsic indignity of permanent unconsciousness than the burdens of unconsciousness.)

In the empty portion of the glass, a suffering, dying patient is legally precluded from hastening death in the most expeditious way possible—namely, by assistance in committing suicide or voluntary active euthanasia. As noted, a patient can die within approximately twenty-one days by resisting bodily intrusions (including manual feeding and artificial nutrition and hydration), but must subsist in a highly debilitated condition for that period. Also, while effective pain relief is an entitlement, law and medicine continue the misguided conventional wisdom that a physician's pure state of mind—meaning specific intention to relieve suffering—is the principal determinant of the legality of risky analgesics. And, of course, not enough healthcare providers have mastered the pain relief techniques now available.

The glass is more empty than full in the sense that while prospective autonomy is a legally accepted principle, its implementation is often denied. Too many healthcare providers choose not to adhere to a patient's advance instructions or to a conscientious surrogate's projection of what course of treatment the now-incompetent patient would have wanted. No effective remedy exists for this behavior, even when a provider has unjustifiably overridden instructions and prolonged the patient's dying process. Numerous jurisdictions have rejected a "wrongful living" damage remedy, reasoning that preservation of life must be an inestimable value surpassing any suffering or indignity that might ensue from an unwanted extension of life.[78] This legal refusal to award damages for a wrongful extension of life ignores that the patient or conscientious surrogate has already determined that the patient is better off dead than alive in the circumstance at hand. This absence of a realistic threat of damages limits the patient or the patient's surrogate to seeking a petition for an injunction or a professional disciplinary action against the provider in question. In addition, an important practical obstacle to implementing a patient's advance instructions is that too many advance directives are so cursory and uninformative about the patient's dignitary values as to be unhelpful to the healthcare providers involved.

The glass appears emptiest with respect to the patchwork of standards that govern surrogate decision making when no clear advance instructions were provided by the now-incompetent patient about his or her medical treatment during the dying process. The articulated approaches—including substituted judgment and best interests—tend to be confused and confusing. They do not adequately acknowledge the common preferences people have regarding dignity in the dying process. Sadly, the glass has least content in states like New York, Michigan, and Wisconsin, where the absence of clear advance instructions can relegate a dying patient to a prolonged dying process characterized by extreme debilitation and indignity, if not suffering.

We've come a long way since *Quinlan* in establishing a legal framework that provides options for preserving a modicum of dignity in the dying process. We have a long way to go.

NOTES

1. *In re Quinlan*, 355 A.2d 647 (N.J. 1976). Death and dying jurisprudence actually predates *Quinlan*, but *Quinlan* was a landmark case. See note 7.

2. See, for example, *Foody* v. *Manchester Memorial Hospital*, 482 A.2d 713 (Conn. 1984); *John F. Kennedy Hospital* v. *Bludworth*, 452 So. 2d 921 (Fla. 1984); In re Severns, 421 A.2d 1334 (Del. 1980).

3. See, for example, *In re Conroy*, 486 A.2d 1209 (N.J. 1985); *In re Torres*, 357 N.W.2d 332 (Minn. 1984); *In re Lydia F. Hall Hospital*, 455 N.Y.S.2d 706 (N.Y. Sup. Ct. 1982).

4. *Cruzan* v. *Director, Missouri Department of Health*, 497 U.S. 261 (1990).

5. *Washington* v. *Glucksberg*, 521 U.S. 702 (1997).

6. *McKay* v. *Bergstedt*, 801 P.2d 617 (Nev. 1990); *In re Farrell*, 529 A.2d 404 (N.J. 1987); *Satz* v. *Perimutter*, 362 So. 2d 160 (Fla. Dist. Ct. App. 1978).

7. A blood transfusion involves a relatively slight physical invasion, but sometimes entails a severe insult to a patient's conscientious religious scruples. In Jehovah's Witnesses' cases predating *Quinlan*, the courts

reached mixed results—sometimes upholding and sometimes rejecting a patient's wish to reject treatment. See N. L. Cantor, "A patient's decision to decline life-saving medical treatment: Bodily integrity versus the preservation of life," *Rutgers Law Review* 26 (1973): 230–36. Post-*Quinlan*, courts have uniformly upheld an adult's prerogative to reject a blood transfusion. See *Public Health Trust* v. *Wons*, 541 So. 2d 96 (Fla. 1989); *Fosmire* v. *Nicoleau*, 551 N.E.2d 77 (N.Y. 1990); C. K. Goldberg, "Choosing life after death: Respecting religious beliefs and moral conventions in near death decisions," *Syracuse Law Review* 39 (1988): 1197–1265.

8. *In re Conroy*, 486 A.2d 1209 (N.J. 1985); *Fosmire* v. *Nicoleau*, 551 N.E.2d 77 (N.Y. 1990); see P. G. Peters, "The State's interest in the preservation of life: From Quinlan to Cruzan," *Ohio State Law Journal* 50 (1989): 891–1010.

9. *Superintendent of Belchertown State School* v. *Saikewicz*, 370 N.E.2d 417 (Mass. 1977); *In re Colyer*, 660 P.2d 738 (Wash. 1983); *Bartling* v. *Superior Court*, 209 Cal. Rptr. 220 (Cal. Ct. App. 1984).

10. J. F. Daar, "A clash at the bedside: Patient autonomy a physician's professional conscience," *Hastings Law Journal* 44 (1993): 1241–95.

11. *Application of Georgetown College*, 331 F.2d 1000 (D.C. Cir. 1964).

12. *Fosmire* v. *Nicoleau*, 551 N.E.2d 77 (N.Y. 1990); *In re Dubreuil*, 603 So. 2d 538 (Fla. Dist. Ct. App. 1992).

13. M. Siegler and A. J. Weisbard, "Against the emerging stream: Should fluids and nutritional support be *discontinued*?" *Arch Int Med* 145 (1985): 129; D. Callahan, "On feeding the dying," *Hastings Center Report* 13 (Oct. 1983): 22.

14. See, for example, *In re Conroy*, 486 A.2d 1209,1236 (N.J. 1985); *Matter of Mary Hier*, 464 N.E.2d 959, 960-65 (Mass. App. Ct. 1984); *Barber* v. *Superior Court*, 195 Cal. Rptr. 484,491-94 (Cal. Dist. Ct. App. 1983).

15. *Satz* v. *Perlmutter*, 363 So. 2d 160, 162 (Fla. Dist. Ct. App. 1978); *Superintendent of Belchertowm State School* v. *Saikewicz*, 370 N.E.2d 417 (Mass. 1977).

16. *Matter of Peter*, 529 A.2d 419, 425 (NJ. 1987); *Thor* v. *Superior Court*, 855 P.2d 375 (Cal. 1993).

17. Compare *Zant* v. *Prevatte*, 286 S.E.2d 715 (Ga. 1982) and *Singletary* v. *Costello*, 665 So. 2d 1099 (Fla. App. 1996), both finding a prisoner's right to hunger strike, with *Laurie* v. *Senecal*, 666 A.2d 806 (R.I. 1995), *In re Caulk*, 480 A.2d 93 (N.H. 1984), and *Van Holden* v. *Chapman*, 450 N.Y.S.2d 623

(N.Y. App. Div. 1982), all rejecting any such right. See S. C. Sunshine, "Should a hunger-striking prisoner be allowed to die?" Note, *Boston College Law Review* 25 (1984): 423–58.

18. For a fuller account of this position, see N. L. Cantor and G. C. Thomas III, "The legal bounds of physician conduct hastening death," *Buffalo Law Review* 48 (2000): 98–107.

19. *In re Brooks* (N.Y. Sup. Ct. 1987), unpublished opinion; *In re Plaza Health and Rehabilitation Center* (N.Y. Sup. Ct. 1984) unpublished opinion; *Matter of Ione Bayer* (N.C. 1987) unpublished opinion. See I. Byock, "Patient refusal of nutrition and hydration: Walking the ever-finer line," *Amer J Hosp Palliat Care* (March 1995): 8; P. Eddy, "A conversation with my mother," *JAMA* 272 (1994): 179.

20. See P. C. Sorum, "Limiting cardiopulmonary resuscitation," *Albany Law Review* 57 (1994): 617–47; "CEJA guidelines for the appropriate use of DNR orders," *JAMA* 265 (1991): 1868.

21. See K. A. Koch, B. W. Meyers, and S. Sandroni, "Analysis of power in medical decision making: An argument for physician autonomy," *Law, Medicine & Health Care* 20, no. 4 (1992): 320–26; N. Jecker, "Knowing when to stop: The limits of medicine," *Hastings Center Report* 21(1991): 5.

22. R. Veatch and C. Spicer, "Medically futile care: The role of the physician in setting limits," *Amer J Law Med* 18 (1992): 15–36; J. Lantos et al., "The illusion of futility in clinical practice," *Amer J Med* 87 (July 1989): 81.

23. See J. Menikoff, "Demanded medical care," *Arizona State Law Journal* 30 (1998): 1091–1130.

24. See Veatch and Spicer, "Medically futile care"; N. L. Cantor, "Can healthcare providers obtain judicial intervention against surrogates who demand 'medically inappropriate' life support for incompetent patients?" *Crit Care Med* 24, no. 5 (1996): 884.

25. *In re Wanglie*, Px-91-283 (4th Judicial District, Hennepin County Minnesota, July 1991).

26. *Gilgunn* v. *Massachusetts General Hospital* (Mass. Superior Court, Suffolk County, April 21, 1995).

27. *Causey* v. *St. Francis Medical Center*, 719 So. 2d 1072 (La. Ct. App. 1998). See also Menikoff, "Demanded medical care," pp. 1125–26.

28. *Velez* v. *Bethune*, 466 S.E.2d 627 (Ga. Ct. App. 1995); *Rideout* v. *Hershey Medical Center* (Pa. Common Pleas 1995) unpublished opinion.

29. *Matter of Baby K.*, 832 F. Supp. 1022 (E.D. Va. 1993), aff'd 16 F.3d 590 (4th Cir. 1994), cert. denied 115 5. Ct. 91 (1994).

30. B. Rich, "A prescription for the pain: The emerging standards of care for pain management," *William Mitchell Law Review* 26 (2000): 1–91; Symposium, "Appropriate management of pain: Addressing the clinical, legal, and regulatory barriers," *J Law, Med Ethics* 24 (1996): 285–421.

31. New York State Task Force on Life and the Law, *When Death Is Sought: Assisted Suicide and Euthanasia in the Medical Context* (New York: New York State Task Force on Life and Law, 1994).

32. S. R. Latham, "Aquinas and morphine: Notes on double effect at the end of life," *DePaul Journal of Health Care Law* 1 (1997): 625; D. C. Thomasma, "Ensuring a good death," *Bioethics Forum* 13, no. 4 (winter 1997): 14.

33. Cantor and Thomas, "The legal bounds of physician conduct hastening death," pp. 126–31.

34. *Washington* v. *Glucksberg*, 521 U.S. 702 (1997); *Vacco* v. *Quill*, 521 U.S. 793 (1997).

35. *Vacco* v. *Quill*, 521 U.S. 793, 808 (1997).

36. *Washington* v. *Glucksberg*, 521 U.S. 702, 780–81 (1997), J. Souter, concurring; id. at 750–52, J. Stevens, concurring; id. at 736–38, J. O'Connor, concurring; id. at 791, J. Breyer, concurring.

37. Cantor and Thomas, "The legal bounds of physician conduct hastening death," pp. 116–20.

38. A. R. Fleischman, "Ethical issues in pediatric pain management and terminal sedation," Commentary, *J Pain Sympt Mgmt* 15 (1998): 261.

39. R. N. Wennberg, *Terminal Choices: Euthanasia, Suicide, and the Right to Die* (Grand Rapids: William B. Eerdsman, 1989), p. 105.

40. D. Orentlicher, "The Supreme Court and terminal sedation: Rejecting assisted suicide, embracing euthanasia," *Hastings Constitutional Law Quarterly* 24 (1997): 947–68; J. Robertson, "Respect for life in bioethical dilemmas—The case of physician-assisted suicide," *Cleveland State Law Review* 45 (1997): 329–43.

41. See also Cantor and Thomas, "The legal bounds of physician conduct hastening death," pp. 145–51.

42. *Compassion in Dying* v. *Washington*, 79 F. 3d 790 (9th Cir. 1996); *Quill* v. *Koppell*, 80 F.3d 716 (2d Cir. 1996).

43. *Washington* v. *Glucksberg*, 521 U.S. 702 (1997); *Vacco* v. *Quill*, 521 U.S. 793 (1997).

44. *Krischer* v. *Mclver*, 697 So. 2d 97 (Fla. 1997); *People* v. *Kevorkian*, 527 N.W.2d 714 (Mich. 1994); *Donaldson* v. *Van de Kamp*, 4 Cal. Rptr. 2d 59 (Calif. Ct. App. 1992).

45. See D. A. Pratt, "Too many physicians: Physician-assisted suicide after Glucksberg/Quill," *Albany Journal of Law, Science & Technology* 9 (1999): 200–201, 233; T. Quill et al., "Care of the hopelessly ill: Proposed clinical criteria for physician-assisted suicide," *N Engl J Med* 327 (1992): 1380.

46. Compare C. Gomez, *Regulating Death: Euthanasia and the Case of the Netherlands* (New York: The Free Press, 1991), opposing physician-assisted suicide, with J. Griffiths, A. Bood, and H. Weyers, *Euthanasia & Law in the Netherlands* (Amsterdam: Amsterdam University Press, 1998), favoring physician-assisted suicide.

47. For example, J. A. Robertson, "Second thoughts on living wills," *Hastings Center Report* 21, no. 5 (November 1991): 6–9; G. McGee, "Paper shields: Why advance directives still don't work," *Princeton Journal of Bioethics* 1, no. 1 (1998): 42–56.

48. R. Dresser, "Confronting the near irrelevance of advance directives," *J Clin Ethics* 5, no. 1 (1994): 55–56; R. Dresser and J. A. Robertson, "Quality of life and nontreatment decisions for incompetent persons," *Law, Medicine & Health Care* 17 (1989): 234–44.

49. This language is from a model used by Choice in Dying, a national organization promoting death with dignity [online], http://www.esinteractrive.com [1 June 2000].

50. N. L. Cantor, "Making advance directives meaningful," *Psychology, Public Policy, and Law* 4 (1998): 646–52.

51. M. J. Lerner, "State natural death acts: Illusory protection of individuals' life-sustaining treatment decisions," *Harvard Journal of Legislation* 29 (1992): 175–221.

52. N. L. Cantor, *Advance Directives and the Pursuit of Death with Dignity* (Bloomington: Indiana University Press, 1993), pp. 48–50; S. M. Wolf, "Honoring broader directives," *Hastings Center Report* 21, no. 5 (September 1991): S8-S9; *Matter of Tavel*, 661 A.2d 1061 (Del.1995). But see *Wright* v. *Johns Hopkins Health Systems*, 728 A.2d 166, 176–79 (Md. 1999); *First Healthcare Corp.* v. *Rettinger*, 467 S.E.2d 243 (N.C. 1996); *HCA* v. *Miller*, #14-98-00582-CV (Tex. Ct. App. 2000), suggesting that statutes such as natural death acts or living will acts provide the exclusive route for removal of life support from now-incompetent patients.

53. *Matter of Westchester County Medical Center*, 531 N.E.2d 607 (N.Y. 1988); *DeGrella v. Elston*, 858 S.W.2d 698 (Ky. 1993); *Mack v. Mack*, 618 A.2d 744 (Md. 1993); *Cruzan v. Harmon*, 760 S.W.2d 408 (Mo. 1988). See also *In re Gardner*, 534 A.2d 947 (Me. 1987). Note, however, that the narrow approaches have been changed by judicial interpretation in Missouri [*Warren v. Wheeler*, 858 S.W.2d 263 (Mo. Ct. App. 1993)] and by statute in Maryland. See D. E. Hoffmann, "The Maryland Health Care Decisions Act: Achieving the right balance?" *Maryland Law Review* 53 (1994): 1064–1135.

54. *Spahn v. Eisenberg*, 543 N.W.2d 485 (Wis. 1997); *In re Martin*, 538 N.W.2d 399 (Mich. 1995).

55. P. Filene, *In the Arms of Others: A Cultural History of the Right to Die in America* (Chicago: Ivan R. Dee, 1998), pp. 109–10.

56. Courts seem to apply the clear and convincing standard with less rigor if the patient is permanently unconscious. See *In re Gardner*, 534 A.2d 947, 952–53 (Me. 1987). Nancy Cruzan herself benefited from this tendency. Upon remand from the Supreme Court, her parents presented additional evidence of her expressed wishes and a trial court authorized the removal of life support. Missouri courts also have interpreted *Cruzan* narrowly, as applying only to removal of artificial nutrition and hydration. See *Warren v. Wheeler*, 858 S.W.2d 263 (Mo. Ct. App. 1993).

57. *Cruzan v. Director, Missouri Dept. of Health*, 497 U.S. 261 (1990).

58. *Superintendent of Belchertown State School v. Saikewicz*, 370 N.E.2d 417, 423 (Mass. 1977); *John F. Kennedy Memorial Hospital v. Bludworth*, 452 So.2d 921 (Fla. 1984); *In re Colyer*, 660 P.2d 738 (Wash. 1983).

59. *In re Fiori*, 673 A.2d 905 (Pa. 1995); *Matter of Tavel*, 661 A.2d 1061 (Del. 1995); *Estate of Longeway*, 549 N.E.2d 292, 299–300 (Ill. 1989); *Brophy v. New England Sinai Hospital*, 497 N.E.2d 626, 631–32 (Mass. 1986).

60. *In re Jobes*, 529 A.2d 434 (N.J. 1987); *In re Fiori*, 673 A.2d 905 (Pa. 1995).

61. M. R. Wicclair, *Ethics and the Elderly* (New York: Oxford University Press, 1993), pp. 56–60; *Estate of Longeway*, 549 N.E.2d 292, 306 (Ill. 1989), J.Ward dissenting.

62. S. G. Pollock, "Life and death decisions: Who makes them and by what standards?" *Rutgers Law Review* 41 (1989): 518–22.

63. *In re Grant*, 747 P.2d 445 (Wash. 1987); *In re Conroy*, 486 A.2d 1209 (N.J. 1985); *In re Rosebush*, 491 N.W.2d 633 (Mich. Ct. App. 1992).

64. See New York State Task Force on Life and the Law, *When Others Must Choose: Deciding for Patients without Capacity* (New York: New York State Task Force on Life and the Law, 1992), p. 55; M. Strasser, "Incompetents and the right to die: In search of meaningful standards," *Kentucky Law Journal* 83 (1995): 778.

65. R. Dresser, "Missing persons: Legal perspectives of incompetent persons," *Rutgers Law Review* 46 (1994): 666–91.

66. Peters, "The State's interest in the preservation of life," p. 942; Strasser, "Incompetents and the right to die," pp. 744–45.

67. President's Commission for the Study of Ethical Problems in Medicine and Biomedical Behavioral Research, *Deciding to Forgo Life-Sustaining Treatment: Ethical, Medical, and Legal Issues in Treatment Decisions* (Washington, D.C.: U.S. Government Printing Office, 1983), pp. 135–36.

68. *Rasmussen v. Fleming*, 741 P.2d 674, 684 (Ariz. 1987); *Barber v. Superior Court*, 195 Cal. Rptr. 484, 493 (Cal. Ct. App. 1983); *In re R.H.*, 622 N.E.2d 1071, 1076 (Mass. App. Ct. 1993), mentioning family interests as a legitimate consideration under a substituted judgment formula.

69. President's Commission, *Deciding to Forgo Life-Sustaining Treatment*, p. 135.

70. See, for example, P. A. Singer et al., "Quality end-of-life care: Patients' perspectives," *JAMA* 281 (1999): 163; J. Lindgren, "Death by default," *Law & Contemporary Problems* 56 (1993): 202.

71. *Rasmussen v. Fleming*, 741 P.2d 674, 688–89 (Ariz. 1987); *Barber v. Superior Court*, 195 Cal. Rptr. 484, 493 (Cal. Ct. App. 1983); *In re Fiori*, 673 A.2d 905, 912 n. 11 (Pa. 1985); *In re Grant*, 747 P.2d 445, 451, 457 (Wash. 1987).

72. N. L. Cantor, "Discarding substituted judgment and best interests: Toward a constructive preference standard for dying, previously competent patients without advance instructions," *Rutgers Law Review* 48 (1996): 1257–72; Lindgren, "Death by default," p. 202.

73. *Superintendent of Belchertown State School v. Saikewicz*, 370 N.E.2d 417 (Mass. 1977); *In re Grant*, 747 P.2d 445 (Wash. 1987). Lindgren, "Death by default," p. 202.

74. M. Danis et al., "Patients and families' preferences for medical intensive care," *JAMA* 260 (1988): 797; D. E. Hoffmann et al., "The dangers of directives or the false security of forms," *J Law Med Ethics* 24 (1996): 10–11; Singer et al., "Quality end-of-life care: Patients' perspec-

tives," p. 163; R. A. Pearlman et al., "Insights pertaining to patient assessments of states worse than death," *J Clin Ethics* 4 (1993): 35.

75. S. H. Kadish, "Letting patients die: Legal and moral reflections," *California Law Review* 80 (1992): 882.

76. Cantor, "Making advance directives meaningful," pp. 646–52.

77. Cantor, "Discarding substituted judgment and best interests," 1265; K. E. Schrode, "Life in limbo, revising policies for permanently unconscious patients," *Houston Law Review* 31 (1995): 1648–53; Lindgren, "Death by default," p. 202; M. Angell, "After *Quinlan*: The dilemma of the persistent vegetative state," *N Engl J Med* 330 (1994): 1524, 1525.

78. *Anderson v. St. Francis Hospital*, 671 N.E.2d 225 (Ohio 1996); M. Strasser, "Wrongful life, wrongful birth, wrongful death, and the right to refuse treatment," *Missouri Law Review* 64 (1999): 29–76; A. Milani, "Better off dead than disabled? Should courts recognize a wrongful living cause of action?" *Washington & Lee Law Review* 54 (1997): 149–228.

CONTRIBUTORS

ANN ALPERS, J.D., Assistant Professor of Medicine, Program in Medical Ethics and the Division of Internal Medicine in the Department of Medicine, University of California, San Francisco.

MARCIA ANGELL, M.D., Senior Lecturer in Social Medicine at the Harvard Medical School and former Editor in Chief, *New England Journal of Medicine*.

LESSIE BASS, D.S.W., Associate Professor, School of Social Work, East Carolina University.

JANET BODELL, S.F.O., R.N., B.S., Spiritual Care Nurse, Riverside Osteopathic Hospital, Trenton, Michigan.

NORMAN L. CANTOR, J.D., Professor of Law and Justice, Nathan L. Jacobs Scholar, Rutgers University School of Law.

BRUCE H. CHAMBERLAIN, M.D., F.A.C.P., Chief Medical Officer, Vista Care Hospice, Scottsdale, Arizona.

KAREN Y. CHAPMAN, M.S.W., East Carolina School of Social Work.

HELEN S. CHAPPLE, R.N., M.A., C.D.E., C.C.R.N., Nurse and Certified Death Educator, Neurological Intensive Care Unit, University of Virginia Health Sciences Center, Charlottesville.

NICHOLAS A. CHRISTAKIS, M.D., PH.D., M.P.H., Professor of Medical Sociology, Department of Health Care Policy, Harvard Medical School.

ELIZABETH C. CLIPP, PH.D., M.S., R.N., Professor in the School of Nursing and Department of Medicine, Division of Geriatrics, Duke University Medical Center.

TAD DUNNE, PH.D., Research Associate at Blue Cross and Blue Shield of Michigan and Editor, *Lonergan Studies Newsletter*.

JOSEPH J. FINS, M.D., Associate Professor of Medicine and Director of Medical Ethics at the New York Weill Cornell Medical Center, New York–Presbyterian Hospital, and Associate for Medicine at the Hastings Center.

N. GREGORY HAMILTON, M.D., Psychiatrist and Spokesperson for Physicians for Compassionate Care, Portland, Oregon.

ANN JACKSON, M.M., Executive Director and Chief Executive Officer, Oregon Hospice Association.

W. CLAY JACKSON, M.D., DIP.TH., Assistant Professor, Department of Family Medicine, Department of Human Values and Ethics, University of Tennessee Health Sciences Center, Memphis.

MARSHALL B. KAPP, J.D., M.P.H., Professor of Community Health and Psychiatry and Director of Geriatric Medicine and Gerontology, Wright State University Medical School.

BARBARA COOMBS LEE, F.N.P., J.D., President and CEO of Compassion in Dying, a nonprofit group supporting the legalization of physician-assisted suicide.

BERNARD LO, M.D., Professor of Medicine and Director of the Program in Medical Ethics at the University of California, San Francisco.

DOUGLAS MACDONALD, M.S.W., C.S.W., Instructor, School of Social Work, Syracuse University.

LAUREN M. MCINTYRE, PH.D., Assistant Professor, Department of Agronomy, Computational Genomics, Purdue University.

MAYA MCNEILLY, PH.D., Adjunct Assistant Research Professor, Division of Medical Psychology, Duke University Medical Center.

CLYDE NABE, PH.D., Faculty Emeritus, Department of Philosophical Studies, Southern Illinois University, Edwardsville.

NAOMI NAIERMAN, M.P.A., President and CEO, American Hospice Foundation.

SALLY NUNN, R.N., Faculty Associate, Center for Bioethics, University of Pennsylvania.

TIMOTHY E. QUILL, M.D., Professor of Medicine, Primary Care Unit, University of Rochester School of Medicine.

SUSAN REDDING, B.S., M.S.N., Clinical Nurse Specialist and End-of-Life Coordinator, Pitt Country Memorial, Greenville, North Carolina.

PAUL ROUSSEAU, M.D., Associate Chief of Staff for Geriatrics and Extended Care, Director of Palliative Care, Veterans Administration Medical Center, Phoenix, Arizona.

MYLES N. SHEEHAN, S.J., M.D., Associate Professor of Medicine and Geriatric Specialist, Stritch School of Medicine, Loyola University, Chicago.

KAREN E. STEINHAUSER, PH.D., Health Services Specialist, Veteran Affairs Medical Center, Durham, North Carolina.

JAMES A. TULSKY, M.D., Veteran Affairs Medical Center, Durham, North Carolina.

MARIE-ANGE WENG, R.N., PH.D., Retired Professor of Nursing and Hospice Education, Madonna University, Livonia, Michigan.